Practice by the Book

A
Christian Doctor's Guide to Living and Serving

Gene Rudd, M.D.
Al Weir, M.D.

SPECIAL GIFT EDITION

Christian
Medical
Association®
Changing Hearts in Healthcare

Practice by the Book
Christian Medical & Dental Associations Resources

Practice by the Book: A Christian Doctor's Guide to Living and Serving
Copyright© 2005 by Christian Medical & Dental Associations

Requests for information should be addressed to:
Christian Medical & Dental Associations
P.O. Box 7500
Bristol, TN 37621

Library of Congress Cataloging-in-Publication Data
Rudd, Gene, 1951-
Weir, Al, 1951-
  Practice by the Book: A Christian Doctor's Guide to Living and Serving
  ISBN 0-970-66314-5
  Library of Congress Control Number: 2005922635

Suggested library cataloging information:
This is a comprehensive look at how biblical principles can and should guide the lives of doctors as they relate to God, family, community, and their professions.

Cover design by Jay Huron. Interior design by David B. Biebel.

Acknowledgements & Notes

We are thankful to God for allowing us to do this project. Our prayer is that he, only, will be glorified through it. Every part that is good, every part that is pure, and every part that is lovely is from him. We will take the blame for the rest.

We also thank the Christian Medical & Dental Associations for entrusting this labor of love to us. (Note: In many places in the text, the initials CMDA are used instead of spelling out the full name of the organization.)

Below are listed the colleagues who contributed sections and chapters. The editing process attempted to glean and distribute the best material throughout the chapters into one voice; therefore, it is not possible to identify each contribution with its author. We are grateful and indebted to each.

David Allen, M.D.

Ruth Bolton, M.D.

Stan Cobb, D.D.S.

Steve Copeland

John Crouch, M.D.

Richard Donlon, M.D.

Patti Francis, M.D.

Curtis Harris, M.D., J.D.

William Howard

Ken Hekman

William Griffin, D.D.S.

Alan Nelson, M.D.

Robert Orr, M.D.

William Peel, Th.M.

Clydette Powell, M.D., M.P.H.

Andy Sanders, M.D.

Steven Sartori, M.D.

David Stevens, M.D., M.A. (Ethics)

David Topazian, DDS

A special "thank you" goes to David Biebel for his editing, design, and advice, and to Sandy Huron for her careful review of the manuscript in its final stages.

And lastly, we wish to thank our families, especially our wives, Becky and Gay, for being gracious to allow us time away from family responsibilities to attend to this project.

Our prayer is that God will use this book to impact you in such a way that you will "Practice by the Book."

Al Weir, M.D.

Gene Rudd, M.D.

CONTENTS

(In addition to the primary authors, chapter contributors are noted below)

CHAPTER 1

What in This World is a Christian Doctor?

W hen I (AW) was a young man, I looked up to my father. I can still remember the smells of antisepsis when I walked the hospital halls with him, reaching up to hold his hand, amazed at this man who touched and healed. He was a man of dignity, intelligence, love—and a man like Christ to me. My goal in life was to be like him, *a Christian doctor.*

Then, one day I became one, a Christian doctor . . . and I was totally lost in direction. I was incredibly successful in my practice from the start, my office and hospital filled with patients whom I was competently serving. But in the rush and burden of practice I was disoriented. I wondered: *What am I really doing for Christ?*

Out of that disorientation, God clearly called and my wife and two children and I followed that call to Eku, Nigeria as medical missionaries. Once I was a missionary, I was confident that I could be a Christian doctor. Those years were the most fun of my medical career. I was needed without a doubt–incredibly interesting diseases everywhere: trypanosomiasis, tetanus, and malaria–patient after patient survived because I was there. We had a gorgeous flame tree in our back yard and a river we would walk to every day after work to wash off the tropical sweat. It was great! And then through an illness, God called us home to Memphis, Tennessee.

It was tough living back here; I was a man who had lost his mission. For years I begged God to send us back to the mission field and he refused. Seven years passed before God released me from that dream and placed another dream in my heart. In those seven years of struggle and prayer God showed me that there was a mission for me in Memphis, Tennessee if I would choose to follow it. That mission was called *becoming a Christian doctor.* I have been pursuing it ever since.

Each step on that mission has been challenging, exciting, uncharted, and dangerous. It is a complicated mission. Each step could have destroyed my effectiveness as a Christian. Each step could have brought a tremendous victory. I have many times faced both victory and defeat.

This book is written so that we may pursue that mission together. Are you willing to try? *Becoming a Christian doctor* is not easy but it's probably why God placed you in medicine or dentistry. If you choose to take on such a mission, many questions will confront you, including:

1. What about money? One of the most powerful forces in the world – if conquered, it can be a tremendous tool for the glory of God. When it conquers us, it leads to greed, self-centeredness, a quest for security outside of God, and financial abuse of our patients.

2. What about time? As Christian doctors, how do we divide time between patients, family, recreation, church, and friends? What will be the most important when we have to choose?

3. What about competence? It is our competence that both eases suffering and validates our voice for God.

4. What about compassion? Our compassion with competence is the very touch of Jesus. How do we keep our compassion out of the brier patch of busyness, money, and fatigue?

5. What about family? Our families should be more precious to us than anything else, other than the Lord himself, and yet doctor after doctor neglects and even loses his/her family.

6. What about devotion? In the midst of tremendous time pressures, how will I as a Christian doctor establish and maintain time alone with God?

7. What about place? Where and who does God want me to serve?

8. What about witness? How do we let our patients know that the love we show them comes from Jesus Christ?

Each of these questions is a mountain to climb in the frontier of the Christian doctor. I have a sign in my office – words of Helen Keller – "Life is a daring adventure or nothing." Just so, becoming a Christian doctor is a daring adventure if we choose to really seek it.

As a practicing oncologist, I see approximately fifty patients a day in my hospital and office and each day I face each of these questions – each day I succeed or fail in these challenges and each night I stand before God with a day I cannot recover. As I face these challenges and work among doctors who are either Christian, Jewish, Muslim, or apathetic about their faith, I ask myself: *What really is the difference between a Christian doctor and all the others?*

All the doctors we know have passed their exams and have moved into the life of treating sick people or teaching others to do so. That is our job, our work; we are doctors. Many who are not Christian are moral, compassionate, and competent. But, something else has happened to us as Christian doctors. At some time in our lives, each of us has come to see that God came to earth in the person of a man called Jesus, and died for our sins, and rose from death to take his rightful place as the Lord of all creation. We saw this truth; we said we would accept his gift of forgiveness and would follow him wherever he led us. This has changed our lives – this has made us Christians. The interesting thing is this: When Christ changed our lives to make us Christians, he also changed the kind of doctors that we should become. What in this world is a Christian doctor? The following five characteristics are distinctive of Christian doctors.

1. Christian doctors have a different understanding of time.

Christian doctors know that life does not last for a few good years and then it is over. Life is everlasting. Often as an oncologist I face the tears of those who have lost someone they loved. If they are Christians, my message to them is: "One of the real tragedies of our lives is that we must be separated from each other for a time before we can be together forever – but we will be together forever, someday soon." Most of us as doctors wish to reduce the suffering of our patients because we love them, but all of us know that all of our patients will die someday. Whether it takes two years with cancer, thirty years with heart disease, or even if it comes in the blinding explosion of a plane crashing into their office building, all of our patients will die.

A patient of mine, Debbie, had breast cancer. One day, as I left her hospital room with great sadness, I wished her well. Sensing my heart, she said to me, "Don't worry doctor. If you don't cure me with your medicines, then God will cure me when I get to heaven." Debbie knew that life is everlasting and Debbie is now alive in heaven with God. As Christian doctors we know that life is everlasting. That does two things for us: (a) it gives us hope when we see our patients dying – life does not have to be over for them; (b) it hands us a challenge – we need to help our patients know God so they can live forever with him.

Christian doctors have a different concept of time.

When Christ changed our lives to make us Christians, he also changed the kind of doctors that we should become.

Reality is science but it is also more than science.

2. Christian doctors have a different understanding of reality.

Many of our colleagues feel that our life, our thoughts, and our dreams are nothing but biochemical reactions, limited by the laws of science . . . that our very lives are biological accidents. I once spoke to a hundred and fifty medical students about stem cell research. "Don't you ever let a professor tell you that you are a biological accident," I said. "You were created by God with a purpose." Unfortunately, many of our colleagues teach that reality is limited to phenomenas that can be proved by science.

A Christian doctor is a good scientist. I believe strongly in the scientific method. I am a clinical professor of medicine at our medical school. However, *I know that there is more to reality than that which we can touch or define by scientific laws.* It was God who created all of the biochemistry that we discover. God allows us as doctors to learn his secrets of science so that we can help people in their suffering. Scientific truth is God's truth.

There is also reality beyond that which science can prove. There is science and there is more than science. There is spiritual power in life beyond our scientific understanding. I first witnessed this spiritual power when I was a year old. I do not remember it but I witnessed it. When I was about that age, my brain began degenerating, turning to water and mush. My parents took me to the best neurosurgeons, the ones who knew the best science. They placed drains in my skull. (My children today like to poke their fingers into the holes in my skull where the doctors drained me when I was a small child.) After all of the best science had been attempted, the doctors gave up and told my parents that I would either die or become a "vegetable." They strongly advised my parents to place me in an institution where I could live out my short life and not disturb the rest of the family. My parents loved me enough to hold onto me.

One day they went on a journey, leaving me with my Aunt Eunice. My aunt took me to her small Christian and Missionary Alliance church. There she and her fellow Christian church members prayed over my little body. My parents returned and saw that I was beginning to heal. I became well and I have remained so from that time of prayer. Reality is science but it is also more than science.

Charlie Hester is a patient of mine. A few years ago, Charlie developed visual problems and for some time these went undiagnosed until it was discovered that he had a lymphoma in his brain. He came to me with brain lymphoma and we did the best scientific medicine, using chemotherapy and radiation therapy. The lymphoma went away and there was hope that Charlie was cured. But then the lymphoma returned in his spine and the meninges around the spinal cord. We had much less hope this time that we could cure Charlie but we did all the right scientific things. We gave him radiation therapy. We gave him chemotherapy in his spinal fluid. We gave him aggressive systemic chemotherapy including high dose chemotherapy and stem cell salvage. We all thanked God as the lymphoma disappeared again and, once again, Charlie had a chance to be cured.

But the lymphoma returned once more. This time, it was in his brainstem. I gave up scientifically on trying to cure Charlie. He had completed all the radiation that he could tolerate. He had received all the chemotherapy that his body could stand, and there was very little left that we could do. I told Charlie the truth and explained to him that we could only help him for a little while.

I'll never forget the day, five years later, as Charlie told me and my Muslim resident, "I came to the realization I had been praying wrong. I had been praying for God to help me tolerate the medicine, to help make the medicine work. At the moment when I knew it was scientifically hopeless, I knew it was time to change my prayer. So then I prayed, "Dear God, you are the Creator of the entire universe. You created this body of mine and you understand all of its parts and understand how it works. Come into my life and make the spots go away." Tears came to my eyes as I heard Charlie tell that story. God had answered that prayer and had healed Charlie beyond my capability as a doctor.

We as Christian doctors must learn to weave together our science and the Spirit of God.

3. Christian doctors have a different understanding of value.

What do we value in our life? There are many things on our list of values. *Time* is certainly precious. We have to arrange the stuff of life in some order so that we can be sure to gain the most valuable things first. We put some things on top of our list, the things that we feel in our heart are the most valuable, for these things are the ones we will most likely achieve.

What is on our list–knowledge, relief of human suffering, caring for our families, material possessions, respect, position, power, physical pleasure? All of these can be good things. The question is: In what order do we place them? There should be a clear difference in the prioritized value list of a Christian doctor and a list of a doctor who does not know Jesus Christ.

Several years ago, our CMDA journal, *Today's Christian Doctor*, told the story of Dr. James Collier, an ophthalmologist who had succeeded in life. He had a priority list that he was pleased with, but God was not on top of

What is your prioritized list of values?

"I would not let anyone take away my cancer if it meant missing this journey into God's love."
—James Collier

that list. Then they discovered his lung cancer. His cancer was removed. He thought he was safe – but, then it returned and he knew he would not be cured. Dr. Collier once again turned to God through Jesus Christ. He took his old value list of possessions, respect, pleasure, and knowledge and exchanged them for a new value list. Dr. Collier said, "I know that Jesus is all I have and all I need." God became so wonderful to him that he said, "I would not let anyone take away my cancer if it meant missing this journey into God's love." Dr. Collier learned that the most valuable thing in life is knowing God.

Augustine said, "You have made me for yourself, oh God. My heart will ever restless be, until it finds its rest in thee."

A young man came to Jesus and fell on his knees before him, "Good Teacher, what must I do to inherit eternal life?" he asked. Jesus said to him, "You know the commandments: Do not murder, do not commit adultery, do not steal, do not give false testimony, do not defraud, honor your father and mother."

"Teacher," the man replied, "all these I have kept since I was a boy."

Jesus looked at him and loved him. "One thing you lack. Go sell everything you have and give to the poor, and you will have treasure in heaven. Then come, follow me."

The man's face fell. He went away sad because he was very rich.

Jesus asked the man to move him up on his value list–above his riches; but the man could not do it. That young man lost the first prize because he could not let go of the third prize.

Dietrich Bonhoeffer died in a Nazi concentration camp because as a minister of Christ he could not stand still before the evil of Nazi Germany. Bonhoeffer wrote, "The only man who has the right to say 'Jesus paid it all' is the man who has left his all to follow him." Both Bonhoeffer and Dr. Collier understood that knowing Jesus was worth it all.

Christian doctors have a different understanding of value in this world.

4. Christian doctors live a life with a mission that is greater than themselves.

Psychiatrist Ernest Becker, wrote in his great book *Denial of Death* that all men and women live in a great dilemma. He said that we all dream of great things. We see beauty. We acquire knowledge of science and history, and we are amazed. We imagine a great future for ourselves. As human creatures, are able to dream these things and, because of these dreams, we are able to rise above the animals as little gods. But the scientific truth is that our dreams can never be fully achieved because we are limited by our biology. If we are gods, Becker says, we are "gods with anuses" and "gods who die." Throughout Becker's book the question is asked, "What worthwhile purpose can man hold onto if his life is limited to the scientific fact that death will take every dream he has and dissolve it into nothingness?"

Christian doctors have a different understanding of time – life is everlasting; a different concept of reality – there is a spiritual world as well as a physical world; a different concept of value – to be with God is better than everything. Because of these understandings, Christian doctors have a different mission in life from those who do not know Christ.

A teacher of the law came up to Jesus and asked him, "Of all the commandments, which is the most important?"

"The most important one," said Jesus, "is this: 'Hear, O Israel, the Lord our God, the Lord is one. Love the Lord your God with all your heart and with all your soul and with all your mind and with all your strength.' The second is this: 'Love your neighbor as yourself.' There is no commandment greater than these."

Within those words lies the mission of all Christian doctors:
1. Know that God is One;
2. Love God with everything that we are;
3. Love our fellow man as much as we love ourselves;
4. Work with God in bringing others to love him as we do.

Jesus lived as a model of that mission for the Christian doctor. Jesus did not wish to die on the cross. In the Garden of Gethsemane he prayed, "Father, all things are possible for you. Take this cup from me, yet, not what I will but what you will." Jesus did not want to die, but he loved God more than life. Jesus was saying, "Whatever you tell me to do with my life, I will do it because you are God." Jesus lived the mission of serving God.

Jesus also lived his life on earth touching and healing because he loved. The reward he received from the people he healed was the pain of the cross. Jesus is a model for our mission in this life.

Christian doctors say:
♦ I am here to obey God, whatever he wants me to do with my life.
♦ I am here to serve people with my skills as a doctor. I am here to ease their suffering because I love them. Like Jesus, I will not limit my service to those who can reward me. I will be a servant to my patients. I will be competent.
♦ Because I love them I will point my patients and colleagues to God through Jesus Christ so that they may live a life that has hope and can last forever.

Christian doctors have a mission in life that is greater than themselves.

Jesus is a model for our mission in this life.

5. Christian doctors have a different relationship with God.

From that moment, my fear of death vanished.

The God of the universe comes to live in our hearts. God is here with us to give us peace in hard times. Peace comes from two things: forgiveness and trust. With forgiveness we can put our past behind us. With trust we can understand that our future is in the hands of a good and powerful God. God is here with us to pick us up when we fall. We are not perfect people. We make mistakes and we fall just like all human beings; but, as Christian doctors, we know that God is here to pick us up.

When I was thirty years old and headed for the mission field, I had a significant faith problem. Though I knew Christ and trusted in his sacrifice for my eternal life, I still would experience nights of fear when I would lie awake in cold sweats, afraid of the infinite nothingness of death.

During that time of mission preparation my wife, Becky, became pregnant with our second child. It was a blessing that turned into a disaster. Becky became so ill that nothing could stop her vomiting. In spite of all the medical care we could access, she wasted away. I would often leave work early and rush home to brush her hair and comfort her . . . one day of suffering at a time. She finally became so weak that I had to carry her in my arms to the bathroom. She slipped into a deep depression and I thought she would die.

During one of our hospital admissions a caring doctor suggested an abortion and we agreed. We were broken. God had not come through and we had no hope. The night before the abortion my father walked into our room. "I know that you may never feel the same about me after I tell you this," he said, "but I tell you because I love you. What you are planning to do is wrong."

He left the room and I fell into Becky's arms. We cried for a long time, but when the tears dried, we resolved to keep our child, no matter the cost. Catherine is now a practicing nurse.

I came away from that experience a different person. I remember falling hopelessly and then landing in the arms of God. I can to this day feel the comfort and strength of those arms.

Something else also happened to me that day. From that moment, my fear of death vanished. It was not a rational change in my mind that pushed the fear away; it just vanished. Somehow from within the comfort and security of the arms of God, I lost access to that fear and it has not returned.

Christian doctors have a different relationship with God. God is here for us with power and peace and a hand to lift us when we fall.

In summary:

♦Christian doctors have a different understanding of time: life is eternal.

♦Christian doctors have a different understanding of reality: life is spiritual as well as physical.

♦Christian doctors have a different understanding of value: knowing God is the greatest thing.

♦Christian doctors have a different mission in life: We are here to love and serve God. We are here to love and serve people. We are sent into the world as God's message of love.

♦Christian doctors have a different relationship with God—we serve a God who brings peace and power into our lives and who picks us up when we fall.

*"I am your Message, Lord. Throw me like a blazing torch into the night, so that all may see and understand what it means to be a disciple."
—Maria Skobstsova*

Each of us must choose whether he or she will be a Christian doctor. I have chosen so for myself. And yet, even as I choose, I struggle. Many days I come home tired, after too many patients and too many meetings, to face a family I love and see too little of. I go to bed wondering what I really did for God that day.

I sometimes get fatigued with all the busyness of life, and sometimes I look at my Christian mission as a burden. And sometimes I hear this voice that says, "Just take care of your own and live the normal life—just take care of your own and live the normal life." Sometimes that sounds good to me.

But as that voice whispers in one ear, the voice of God whispers in the other—and I know that I am a Christian doctor and I must not settle for normal life.

Sometimes it helps to have a battle cry that drowns out the voice of the world. I have chosen one for my life. It came from the heart of a woman named Maria Skobstsova, who lived and died in the twentieth century. She had a family—three daughters. She could have sought normal life but she heard the whisper of God and she dedicated her life to caring for refugees on the streets of Paris. She died in a German concentration camp for attempting to rescue the Jews of Paris. Maria Skobstsova knew who she was and knew her reason for being. She once said, "I am your Message, Lord. Throw me like a blazing torch into the night, so that all may see and understand what it means to be a disciple."

Some time ago I went to my farm, where I'm trying to grow fruit trees on a small ridge between two fields. This ridge is separated from the forest on either side by thirty yards of grass, safe from the kudzu vines that are devouring the forest. When I reached my trees I discovered with horror that the kudzu had somehow sensed their presence and had crawled across the

Our mission at CMDA is for you and for me and thousands of others—ordinary doctors in a crazy world, yet willing to take a stand day after day and show the world that we are Christian doctors.

grass and was wrapping itself around those trees. I spent two hours cutting and unraveling the vines that choked my trees. That choking parallels the story of our lives. The individual world of many doctors is complex and heavy—and normal life is wrapping its vines around them—like the kudzu around my fruit trees in Tennessee.

I challenge you to break away. I challenge you to follow the whisper of God and the battle cry of Maria Skobstsova:

"I am your Message Lord. Throw me like a blazing torch into the night so that all may see and understand what it means to be a disciple."

If ever our world needs Christian doctors to adopt this battle cry, it is now.

Our mission in CMDA is not a mission for Bristol, Tennessee, alone. It is a mission for you and for me and thousands of others—ordinary doctors in a crazy world, yet willing to take a stand day after day and show the world that we are Christian doctors.

THREE QUESTIONS TO ASK YOURSELF
1. What goals for my profession have I placed above that of becoming a Christian doctor?
2. Which questions on the second page of this chapter do I most need God's help answering?
3. From what influences or pressures do I need to break away in order to become the doctor God created me to be?

THREE ACTIONS TO CONSIDER
1. Write a mission statement for your life, starting with: "With the life God has given me, I believe he wants me to . . . ."
2. List the possessions, activities, or persons that you value most in life. Every morning, for one week, offer them back to God to use that day for his purpose.
3. Assuming that you as a Christian doctor are God's message, write down what you think the world reads when watching your life?

PRAYER

My God,
You are so great and I am so small. I wonder that you notice me at all, let alone allow me to carry a sword and march beside you to redeem the world. Bend me; break me; mold me; use me. Create in me a servant worthy to be called a Christian doctor.

—Amen

CHAPTER 2

Our Spiritual Foundation

I was leafing through an old photograph album when my gaze was fixed on a long-forgotten photo. It was my picture, standing side by side, arms on shoulders, with a classmate and close friend—two young men together, excited about life and the prospects ahead. We were sharing the same road into life and were eagerly awaiting the fruits of our labors. From the moment of that photo we each progressed through training and on to our careers and to our new families.

That photograph, if taken today, would be changed by more than our ages. Tragically, now there would be only one person in that picture. My friend committed suicide some years ago. When that photo was taken, our individual concern for spiritual life was being drowned out by the fresh excitement of medicine, the hard work at hand, the goals and the rewards that lay ahead. Looking back on the picture, I realize that the deeply buried spiritual questions were the questions that really mattered.

–Andy Sanders, M.D.

Each of us shares a small fragment of life on earth and each of us is trying to build a life worth living. Billions have gone before us, but now is our particular moment in the endless stream of humanity. Whether we pay attention to it or not, we are building our lives, one day at a time, one event at a time, one decision at a time.

Someday, when we look back at the completed work of our days, what will we see? Someday, when we finally see the face of God, what will he say? His words to us that day will depend on two things: the first, an act on the cross; the second, our response to that act.

The action of Christ on the cross is foundational. Nothing else we say in this book (and absolutely nothing we do with our lives) matters were it not for that act in which Jesus, the Son of God, which made provision

The deeply buried spiritual questions were the questions that really mattered.

for the forgiveness of our sins. *"We all, like sheep, have gone astray, each of us has turned to his own way; and the LORD has laid on him the iniquity of us all"* (Isa. 53:6).

God has offered that act, so costly to him, as a free gift to us so that we may be brought back from our sin into the arms of the holy God who loves us. Unless we believe in that action of Christ and choose to follow the Christ who died for us, we have no hope of satisfaction in this life or hope beyond the death we all face. Do not read another page in this book before you ask Jesus Christ to enter your life, to be the sacrifice for your sin, and to be the Lord of your life.

Once God's act and your response to his action are imbedded forever in your soul, you are saved from death, the penalty of sin. You will then live forever with God in heaven–but you will not necessarily live out this present life with any purpose, power, or peace. Being saved for God's kingdom does not necessarily make you live like a citizen of heaven. God loves you enough to die for you and bring you to heaven even if you never live for him, but he created you for far more than that. He created you to become his soldier, to fight beside him as he retakes his kingdom from Satan. He, therefore, gives us a second and continual choice in this life after our salvation–whether we will join him in his battle.

We could sit back and just let life happen, simply let our lives flow with the world. Why not? Is the life the world wants for us really that much different from that taught in Scripture? Aren't they quite similar? A worldly life can be filled with good works, charity, kindness, and other Christian attributes. Of course it can; but good works and honorable attributes are not the ultimate goals in God's plan for our lives. They are but the secondary results of God's best plan–for us to be transformed into his likeness and to work beside him to redeem this world. We can be good doctors and good people without that transformation, but we cannot honor God. We each have a choice to make. It's like choosing between two sides of the curtain:

I was a fourth year medical student. I was beginning to find myself confidant and capable taking care of patients. I remember enjoying the responsibility that I had been given to perform a neurological exam on a young man who was newly quadriplegic. I introduced myself and began my doctor's duties. With a sense of pride, I began my exam, and my "care" of this patient. I was just now beginning to do what I had trained for. This was medicine as I had been taught it, and I was excited to be at the start of my career. As I began using my newly-learned skills on the patient, an older gentleman dressed in a suit entered the room. I barely noticed him, but he soon became one of the most important teachers I have ever had in medicine. He walked to the bed next to my patient's, where another young quadriplegic patient lay and he pulled the curtain. I returned my attention to my work. As I progressed with my questions and exam I could hear the visitor on the other side of the curtain. He began asking his young patient about his view of God. As I progressed down my neurological exam, I heard the suited man progress down the loving plan of God's redemption. My pride in my own efforts and my abilities to care for my patient were quickly slipping away. A special work of true caring and true healing was taking place in that room, but it was not on my side of the curtain. As I was finishing the last few reflexes of my exam, I heard the gentleman ask the young man if he would like to pray and receive Christ into his life as Lord and Savior. As I was closing up my stiff black bag I heard the young man pray and begin eternal life with his loving Creator. I left different from when I came—contemplative now instead of confidant, humbled instead of proud. I had just experienced for the first time medicine on "the other side of the curtain." This was medicine as ministry, in the name of the Lord and in the power of his Spirit; medicine where much more than just flesh and organs are cared for.

–Andy Sanders, M.D.

Each of us, in this moment of time, is building a life. On which side of the curtain are you?

Each of us, in this moment of time, is building a life. *On which side of the curtain are you?* The world would have you stay on the first side and build a good life, but there is a rich life on the other side of the curtain that the Lord has prepared for each of us, a life he wants to use for his eternal purposes. That's where our abundant joy and delight will be found. But how do we build such a life? How can we become the persons that God envisioned when we were knit together in our mothers wombs? (Ps. 139:13)

There are four steps to becoming the people God created us to be. We have already discussed three:

1. Understand where we started, "...for all have sinned and fall short of the glory of God" (Rom. 3:23).
2. Believe to the depth of our souls how we as Christians have come this far, "For the wages of sin is death, but the gift of God is eternal life in Christ Jesus our Lord" (Rom 6:23).
3. Realize our eventual goal, "I want to know Christ and the power of his resurrection and the fellowship of sharing in his sufferings, becoming like him in his death, and so, somehow to attain to the resurrection from the dead" (Phil. 3:10-11).

*God
uses
prayer
as
a way
to
bring
us
to
himself.*

The final step to becoming the people God has created us to be is the most difficult for us to accomplish, and yet, it is filled with the purpose, peace, and power we all seek in this life. This final step is to walk the Path. Walking God's Path is the subject of this book; it involves very practical issues in our daily lives. But walking the practical Path for God in this world demands that we keep "one foot in heaven." We cannot please God with any practical success if we are not spiritually well grounded.

Those of us raised in the church know what it takes to be spiritually well-grounded. If we are seeking to walk God's path in this world we need to deeply commit to four spiritual disciplines:

1. Prayer
2. Bible study
3. Fellowship
4. Worship

These four spiritual disciplines are our signposts and our nutrition as we walk God's path for our individual lives in this world. They are our banners, our shields, and our swords we use to fight beside and for our King to redeem his world. Do you use them well?

PERSONAL PRAYER

All people pray. As doctors who seek to accomplish God's purpose for our lives, how well do we pray? What about the sincerity of our prayers? Does prayer really matter?

Nehemiah was a man faced with great uncertainty. He wanted to faithfully live for God but was unsure of his next step. He thought he was to build the wall around Jerusalem but did not know how to proceed. Nehemiah 1 records for us the next step he took: he prayed. Not a short sentence prayer or two–he labored in prayer. He prayed and fasted for three months! Then God showed him how to proceed.

Prayer was clearly not casual or optional in Daniel's life. Nor did it bring him an easy life. We all remember Daniel's faithfulness in prayer that led him into the lion's den. In Daniel 9 and 10 we see Daniel's heart for prayer. He fasted and prayed for twenty-one days. It was after such patience and persistence in prayer that the angel came to Daniel with words from God.

I was attending a medical conference in Boston a number of years ago. It was there, in my hotel room during a time of Bible study, that I was struck with a most unusual sense that the Lord had something new for my family and me. Little did my wife know what I was about to confront our family with when she greeted me at the airport. A year of questions followed, with uncertainty, but with prayer. We invited two other couples to join us monthly to pray for the Lord's clear guidance. Late night prayer with the family asleep became a common activity. I struggled to know how the Lord wanted me to lead my family.

Slowly my wife and I became aligned, and slowly we loosened our grip on our comfortable and settled life. Late one night, after a year of uncertainty and seeking the Lord in prayer, I was filled with a clear understanding and a settled peace about our future. We have since sold our home and I have cut back my days in the office so that I can minister regularly to my colleagues and residents. Life has changed; we have less stuff and we need less stuff. Sometimes it's hard; but, looking back, we have seen the Lord work wonderfully, and we have no doubt that this has been his plan for us. We simply had to discover that plan through patient and persistent prayer.

–Andy Sanders, M.D.

There are so many scriptural lessons about prayer that we can gain by studying God's Word and listening to our church pastors, but the most important lesson we need to learn about prayer is that God uses prayer as a way to bring us to himself; therefore, he wants our whole heart as we come. Many of us, as we look back on the great times of struggle in our lives, can see a definite correlation between the degree to which our heart poured into our prayers and the discovery of God's favor within those prayers. God honors the tears of those who love him and come to him. We are to pray in faith; we are to pray in private; we are to pray in fellowship; we are to pray continually; but, most of all, we are to pray with our whole hearts.

How do we turn our whole-hearted intentions into practical praying? Let me offer you some suggestions, from experience and from the Scriptures:

1. Set aside regular time to speak with the Lord.
2. Come to him each day with a thankful heart: thankful for your life, your new life with him, his sacrifice, your blessings, those you love, the purpose and the plan that he has created for you.
3. Hand the Lord your sins and refuse to take them back.
4. Give the Lord your dreams and ask him to remold them according to his pleasure.
5. Hand the Lord your plans and let him change them if he wishes
6. Trust the Lord with all you have and with those you love.
7. Listen as you pray; seek his direction throughout your day.

We are to pray in faith; we are to pray in private; we are to pray in fellowship; we are to pray continually; but, most of all, we are to pray with our whole hearts.

Is your
Bible truly
essential
to your life,
or a hammer
that you use
for only
really big
nails?

Each day, in your early morning prayers, consider offering to the Lord of the universe–

All you are,
All you have,
All your dreams,
All your plans,
All your sins,
All those you love.

BIBLE STUDY

What about the Word of God? All of us would state without hesitation that it is indeed essential for building a life for God. But, if someone observed your day, your week, or your year, would they see that the Bible is truly essential to the life you are building, or would they see the Bible as an optional or superficial part of your life–a hammer on the shelf that you choose to bring down for only really big nails?

I have had the privilege these past twelve years of seeing many men, including quite a few busy and established doctors, become transformed in some of the most remarkable ways. Men who had been quite content with their self-directed lives and religious involvement are now excited about the Lord in ways they had never known before. A desire for a comfortable self-run life has now been replaced with a desire for a surrendered, God-glorifying life, and hunger for worldly treasures has been replaced with a hunger for God himself.

How did these remarkable changes take place? It actually only required one simple change in their lives. These men began to study the Bible daily. Twelve years ago a group of us started a Bible study for men. Today over three hundred men attend weekly, eager to learn and to follow the Lord. The changes observed have been truly incredible . . . changes in personal lives, in marriages, and in families. It has all been because of Bible study as a priority in their lives.

I sometimes think back to a physician I invited to the study when we first started. Quite affluent and known for making excellent investments, he turned down my invitation, deciding it wasn't something he needed. Twelve years have passed and his life is quite shattered. I think back to that day when he turned down the offer to study God's Word . . . surely the worst investment decision he has ever made.

–Andy Sanders, M.D.

Does God care whether or not his Word is alive in our hearts? Let's see:

*Isa. 40:8 tells us that we have the privilege of investing ourselves in one thing that will never change or fade. All that we hold and enjoy in this world will one day wither, fade, and disappear except for the Word of God, which will remain unchanged forever.

*Deut. 8:3 says that the Word of God is to be as essential to our life as our physical bread.

*Deut. 11:18 commands us to lay up God's words in our heart and in our soul and to teach these truths continuously to our children, speaking of God's word throughout our life with them.

*1 Pet. 2:2 says we are to desire his Word as a newborn child craves milk. It is to be a consuming and constant desire that will settle for nothing less than to be satisfied with nourishment from the word of God.

*2 Tim. 2:15 says we are to diligently study God's Word and are to never be unprepared and ashamed when called upon to use it.

*David, the man after God's own heart, had a heart for the Word of God. David said that God's ordinances are "more precious than gold, than much pure gold" (Ps. 19:10); "I have hidden your word in my heart that I might not sin against you" (Ps. 119:11); "Your word is a lamp to my feet and a light for my path" (Ps. 119:105); "I open my mouth and pant, longing for your commands" (Ps. 119:131); "...for I delight in your commandments because I love them" (Ps. 119:47); "The law from your mouth is more precious to me than thousands of pieces of silver and gold" (Ps. 119:72); "Oh, how I love your law! I meditate on it all day long" (Ps. 119:97).

Our goal and pursuit is to know Christ more fully and to follow him on his path for us in this life.

Does your daily use of time reveal that God's Word is truly a valued tool in building your life? How might the Lord be calling you to a deeper and more disciplined daily involvement in his holy Word? Is there a Bible study that you should join? Is God calling you to give up sleep in order to read his Word? Is there a competing passion that pulls your time away from his Word? Are there changes to make at home to make it clear to your spouse and children that the Word of God is indeed central in your life and in your passions? Again, here are some simple suggestions:

1. Set aside a definite time to read God's Word each day. Start with fifteen minutes followed by prayer.

2. Read Scripture everyday with your spouse and children. A single verse can change both your life and their lives with God's touch.

3. Meet every week to study God's Word with a small group.

*Is the
Lord
calling
you
to a
deeper
and
more
disciplined
daily
involvement
in his
holy
Word?*

FELLOWSHIP WITH BELIEVERS

Our lives are so busy. Extra time is something we haven't had for many years, perhaps decades. Any spare moment therefore is carefully guarded. We are told by God to spend time in fellowship with other believers and we take that more as a suggestion than a requirement.

How much does God value this area of our lives?

- 1 John 1:7: "...if we walk in the light, as he is in the light..." we will have fellowship with other believers. If we are walking as we ought, fellowship is unavoidable. The true way is narrow, and as we walk in it we will find ourselves in close communion with other pilgrims for Christ.
- Prov. 27:17 and Eccl. 4:11-12: We are to be a faithful brother or sister to other believers. We are told that we sharpen each other's countenance as iron sharpens iron, and that we will be stronger with other believers than we can ever be on our own.
- John 13:35: The world must know that we are Christ's disciples, not by our Bible knowledge, or by our correct doctrine, or by our teaching, or by our deeds, but by our love for other Christians.
- 1 Pet. 1:22: We are to love other Christians fervently. We sometimes think of using that adverb in regard to our love for God, but it's quite challenging to apply that to other believers.
- Heb. 10:24-25: Think, and plan, and be intentional in our stirring up one another to love and good works. We are to be faithful to meet together and to exhort one another.

There is no easy way to be involved in the lives of other Christians. At the same time, there is no way around these commands. God won't change the rules for us because we are busy professionals. Fellowship must play an important role in our lives. If we neglect it, God doesn't offer us an alternative.

I know two doctors who have sought to obey these verses in each other's lives. To do so they have met once a week from six to seven in the morning for the past three years. They have spurred each other on to a level of faithful surrender to their Lord that they could not have achieved on their own. Their personal lives, ministries, and practices have all significantly changed during these years of commitment to each other. Both have now become involved in foreign missions. Their practice offices have also changed significantly. Ministry within their own practices has grown as they have challenged each other to more faithfully serve the Lord.

It may not be clear to us how we can find the time, but the scriptural command to do so remains crystal clear. When the commitment exists, the time will be found. Some time ago we started ten fellowship groups for physicians. These are small groups of three doctors who have made a decision to commit to each other's walk with the Lord. They are now meeting weekly, encouraging each other to remain faithful in service to the Lord. A few months ago none of these doctors had any spare time, but now that they have made this commitment, the time has been made as well.

–Andy Sanders, M.D.

Is fellowship with other believers a divine command or just a suggestion?

Dr. Howard Hendricks loved to share from Ecclesiastes 4:12: "A cord of three strands is not quickly broken." Dr. Hendricks said that these three strands are the kinds of people we need in our lives. First, we all need a "Paul," a person of wisdom, someone with knowledge who is willing to invest time to build into our lives. Second, we all need a "Barnabas," someone to walk beside us and encourage us, someone in whom we can confide and with whom we can grow. Third, we all need a "Timothy," someone in whom we can invest our lives and build into and bring along.

When I became an active member of my church, the "Paul" in my life was six or seven years my junior. He was the pastor of our church. His life was so busy that it was hard for him to make time for me. I decided to close my office on Fridays, the day he usually drove to Amarillo to make hospital rounds, so I could travel with him. The hour and a half going and coming back was a great time of growth for me. I gave up one day of work each week for discipleship.

A fellow doctor could have been my "Barnabas" but there were none in my town. So a cattle rancher became my Barnabas. He was my encourager. To this day, Frank Wilmeth of the Wilmeth Cattle Company is one of my best friends. I can count on him when I need a word to keep me going.

I was blessed by more than one "Timothy." I had six or seven young married men who wanted to learn and grow. I stayed only a step or two in front of them. This diverse group included a yuppie accountant, a working cowboy, a company accountant, a farmer/rancher, and a teacher. I had no idea of the impact the Lord had in these young men's lives through me. When I announced I was leaving, they gave testimonies to what the Lord had done in their lives through me. Their mentoring may have been the only significant thing I left behind when I moved to take a teaching position and attend seminary. Today, I am surrounded by other Timothy's, all medical and dental students.

–Stan Cobb, D.M.D.

Christian fellowship is essential if we are to become the people God created us to be and to accomplish the purpose for which God created us. If

*Christian
fellowship
is
essential
if we are
to become
the persons
that God
created
us to be
and to
accomplish
the purpose
that God
created us
for in
this life.*

we are in fellowship with other believers, we need to evaluate the quality of that fellowship; we must understand that it is not only the practice of fellowship that is important; our spirit of fellowship is critical. That spirit should include sacrifice, acceptance, and grace.

I took a class one semester in which each session began with scenes from a popular television show. Many of the students had never seen "Cheers." After each short clip, we would discuss the positive and negative aspects of the situations. The cast of "Cheers" was a cross-section of society that might be found in such a setting.

Remember the following characters—Sam, the superficial bar owner, a has-been sports figure, ex-alcoholic, interested in women, cars, and his looks; Norm, the likeable, lazy, beer sipping, unemployed accountant; Carla, an uneducated waitress, single mother with a caustic personality; Cliff, a know-it-all postman who lives with his mother; Woody, a naïve, dumber-than-dirt Indiana farm boy with high morals; and, Dr. Frazier Crane, a highly intelligent, exquisitely trained Ivy League medical doctor who is surprised that he finds community with this diverse bunch of people. They are troubled, flawed, seemingly hopeless people who all see themselves as normal. Their lives intertwine and they share genuine community, but not perfect community, as captured by the show's theme song: "Making your way in the world today takes everything you've got. Taking a break from all your worries sure would help a lot. Wouldn't you like to get away? Sometimes you want to go where everybody knows your name, and they're always glad you came. You want to be where you can see our troubles are all the same. You want to be where everybody knows your name."

The discussion in our study group was always lively with laughter. Most of us found some level of identity with the characters. We were impressed with the amount of grace they granted each other. We learned something about community and something about grace and we discovered the diversity that can coexist, especially under the divine mandates of God and the empowerment by his Spirit (John. 13:34, 35).

God demands that we do not live our lives in isolation, but in fellowship. That fellowship is with people who are different from us because God has planned it that way. We are different people who serve different functions, all united in God's business of redeeming the world. If the folks on "Cheers" can get it, we should be able to get it: If we were all alike, life would be boring and God's work through the church would be ineffective. Diversity is God's plan; we should embrace it.

I think I understand even more about the church since the birth of my second daughter, Grace. She was born a bit early, was delivered by an emergency C-sec-

tion ninety miles away from our home at Northwest Texas Hospital in Amarillo, Texas, in February 1985. My wife was in the hospital recovering. Our baby was in the neo-natal unit. I had a new practice to juggle, and a nineteen-month-old daughter, Catie . . . and we experienced grace. Our church came to the rescue in our frantic struggle, and it was so much more than food and help. I came to understand the meaning of Acts 2:42,43: "and they were continually devoting themselves to the apostles' teaching, and to fellowship, to the breaking of bread, and to prayer, and everyone kept feeling a sense of awe" (NASB). Our church didn't meet our needs because of who they were or what we could do for them. They met our needs because of who God is and what he had done in their lives individually and corporately as the church. I experienced grace as a part of the Lord's church, and I never was the same. My wife and I were so touched by what had happened to us that we named our daughter Grace.

–Stan Cobb, D.M.D.

If the folks on "Cheers" can get it, we should be able to get it: If everyone were like me, life would be boring and God's work through the church would be ineffective.

Are you growing and sharing within a Christian community in the way that God has planned for the life of his church? We fool and flatter ourselves if we think we can accomplish anything of significance for Christ without the church beside us to encourage, support, and guide. Paul understood our ineffectiveness as solo Christians when he wrote to the people of Ephesus, encouraging them to work together "...until we all reach unity in the faith and in the knowledge of the Son of God and become mature, attaining to the whole measure of the fullness of Christ. Then we will no longer be infants, tossed back and forth by the waves, and blown here and there by every wind of teaching and by the cunning and craftiness of men in their deceitful scheming. Instead, speaking the truth in love, we will in all things grow up into him who is the Head, that is, Christ. From him the whole body, joined and held together by every supporting ligament, grows and builds itself up in love, as each part does its work" (Eph. 4:13-16). Some doctors may think that this passage was not written for men and women of their stature, but even they must follow it or fail.

Here are some practical suggestions as you seek fellowship with your brothers and sisters in Christ:

1. Make it a priority–near the top of your list–because most that follows on your list is dependent on it.
2. Write down the names of three doctors with whom you desire to pray. Call them until one of them agrees to meet with you at least once.

My wife and I were so touched by what had happened to us that we named our daughter Grace.

3. After you meet and pray, set up a firm date for the next meeting and begin to discuss a regular meeting.
4. At the next meeting decide whether others on your list should be added to your group. Begin to discuss the format of your meeting: time, Bible study, prayer, accountability for witness and pursuit of holiness, search for mission. Mold it around your specific needs as two doctors in God's hands.

WORSHIP

My earliest recollections of church were as a boy in a fellowship outside of Fort Worth, Texas. It was a small country church and my experiences there shaped much of my life to come. My brother and I joked that the best barometer for the sermon was how bad we felt upon leaving–the worse we felt, the better the sermon. Picture a handkerchief wielding, pulpit slapping man drenched in perspiration. Picture a sermon called "Journey through Hell," the light bulbs above the pulpit changed to red. I can't remember what I thought about hell afterward, but I sure knew how I felt about the worship service. I didn't want to go back.

Dr. John Patrick, founder and President of Augustine College, was raised in working-class Birmingham, England and had quite the opposite experience. The sermons he experienced were so benign and dull that he read books during worship and told the preacher as much. It is safe to say that neither of us worshiped.
–Stan Cobb, D.M.D.

The worship of God is sometimes difficult not just for those of us living in the first part of the twenty-first century, but throughout the ages. Ultimately, worthwhile worship happens when we human creatures acknowledge the One God worthy of utter, absolute, irrevocable devotion (Rom. 1:20; Ps. 29:2). Worship of God is the acknowledgement of who God is: the Creator of all, the Sustainer of all, the Redeemer of all, the One who was, who is, and who will return. God is the Alpha and Omega (Rev. 1:8). When we worship, we come into the presence of God in a way that we cannot by any other means. If we find ourselves needing love, we will feel it best when we love him in worship. If we need the reassurance of forgiveness, it is most evident when we worship. If we need direction, his hand is most visible when we worship. If we need peace from a world that would deny his victory, he will most likely lay it across our shoulders when we worship.

Most of us worship best when we gather with fellow believers in our local churches. Though some of our personalities may make it pleasant for us to worship alone, God's presence is usually more evident during corporate worship; and he demands that we come together as a body of believers to seek him and to honor him. The temptations we feel to escape to the lake and the mountains are valid occasionally, but cannot be regular excuses to avoid our responsibility as children of the king to gather with our family and worship our Father.

Having said all of this about worship and fellowship, what responsibilities do we have as doctors within our local churches? Here are a few:

1. Attend regularly. We have many opportunities as affluent adults to spend our Sundays elsewhere, but God has placed us within our local churches for our benefit, for the benefit of our fellow believers, and for the work of his kingdom. We may be able to worship God in nature or at a football game, but he has called us to worship corporately and we will never do it well if we don't do it his way.
2. Give sacrificially. To those who have been given much, much is required. Our giving tells God where our hearts lie and it may be the key to the door of greater service to our Lord of the cross.
3. Worship sincerely. When we worship apathetically, we miss God's presence. Others observe and follow our lead.
4. Offer insight. Each of us experiences God's truth in our lives as he enters our daily existence. The Church exists in part so that we may share those bits of truth with each other. We need to do so regularly in a small group setting.
5. Help guide our churches in carrying out God's redemptive work. The church's business is to complete the work of Christ in saving the lost, in helping to mold Christians to be like Jesus, and in caring for the poor and broken. The local church needs its doctors as leaders in that work. Henry Blackaby in his *Experiencing God* series says, "Look around, see where God is working and come in and work where he is working."
6. Teach, if God so leads. Because of our educational background, many doctors are gifted teachers. Teaching takes time, however; and time is a valuable commodity for most doctors. So, teach if God calls but listen instead if he does not.

God has placed each of us within a local church to play our part in drawing the world to the Father they have left. Few of us are called to be lonely warrior heroes–that's a dream of vanity. Let's get it right and take our place within the community he has called us to.

Prayer, God's Word, fellowship, and worship: These are our signposts and our sources of strength for the path that Christ has bid us follow.

Worship of God is the acknowledgement of who God is: the Creator of all, the Sustainer of all, the Redeemer of all, the one who was, who is, and who will return.

*Our giving
tells
God
where our
hearts lie
and it
may
be the
key
to the door
of greater
service
to our
Lord of
the cross.*

Comfortable, conforming Christianity does not require the use of such. We can build quite a nice Christian life without them. But true, life-changing, kingdom-building, God-glorifying Christianity cannot be lived without them. They are absolutely essential, and much more so than most of us have probably yet realized. Christian doctors have a choice: We can take hold of these spiritual disciplines and walk the path God created us to follow; or we can pretend we are on the path while we play checkers with our friends in prison.

I was recently in Moldova, in Eastern Europe, leading a medical mission team. In a prison courtyard there I was struck with a portrait of our Christian lives. As I looked out upon the faces of hardened men, everything from their expressions, to their tattered clothes, to the guards, to the walls and razor wire spoke clearly to what they were: prisoners. There was no confusion on this point. They were prisoners, walled in from freedom and joys. It was likewise clear who we were. We were free people, there to minister to them and to demonstrate and proclaim to them the gospel of Christ. Our lives were not confined within those walls. Imagine how ridiculous it would have been if, when we were leaving, some of the prisoners had called out to us that we should stay, suggesting that we were one of them and that this prison was our home also. How even more ridiculous it would have been for someone in our group to believe that lie and sit down with them, choosing a life in their prison while the rest of the team left the enclosure.
–Andy Sanders M.D.

That scene is strikingly similar to our lives each day. Each day as we leave for work, we enter the courtyard of this world where prisoners dwell. These prisoners are our colleagues, patients, and friends. They are prisoners to sin, with their lives walled in by the boundaries of this world. We are not the same. We are not walled in by the things that contain them. Our lives are grounded in heaven, in Christ our foundation. We are people of the Way, not prisoners of the world. We have a path to follow, a path meant to free those imprisoned by this world. How foolish to think that some of these prisoners call out to us the lie that we belong with them, that this is our home, and that we share the same goals and purposes they do. How much more foolish that some of us believe them. Some of us actually join with them in this world, settle down with them, and share their goals and pursuits.

We do not belong! Our foundation is not in this world and our boundaries are not the boundaries of this world. Our goal and pursuit is to know Christ more fully and to follow him on his path for us in this life. What a tragic thing when a Christian, believing the lies of this world, settles down and builds his life on a worldly foundation. To avoid this greatest tragedy of any Christian's life we must:

1. Understand where we started: "...for all have sinned and fall short of the glory of God" (Rom. 3:23).
2. Believe to the depth of our souls how we as Christians have come this far: "For the wages of sin is death, but the gift of God is eternal life in Christ Jesus our Lord" (Rom. 6:23).
3. Realize our eventual goal: "I want to know Christ and the power of his resurrection and the fellowship of sharing in his sufferings, becoming like him in his death, and so, somehow, to attain to the resurrection from the dead" (Phil. 3:10).
4. Take hold of God's spiritual disciplines: prayer, Bible study, fellowship, and worship. Take them as our swords and shields, our signposts and our strength; take them and follow the path of Christ for which each of us has been created.

We are people of the Way, not prisoners of the world.

THREE QUESTIONS TO ASK YOURSELF
1. What is the personal foundation of my life, from which I launch out and do all things important?
2. Of the four spiritual disciplines: prayer, Bible study, fellowship, and worship, which one do I accomplish the least well?
3. Have I settled down comfortably in the prison of the secular?

THREE ACTIONS TO CONSIDER
1. Read once a week for a month the Gospel of Luke and focus on the person of Christ, his manner, his actions, and his love.
2. Decide what treasure of this world you need to release so that your hands can better grasp God's tools for building your life in him. Write down the steps necessary to do so.
3. Add one day a month in your schedule to be spent in Christian fellowship, where you ask each other, "What struggle are you having this month in living out God's mission for your life?"

PRAYER

Dear Father,
I am so far from the work you have started to complete in me. Show me how to grasp your tools and then, please use them to fashion me into your likeness. Anything less is not enough.

—Amen

CHAPTER 3

Character

"What you are stands over you the while, and thunders so that I cannot hear what you say to the contrary."

—Ralph Waldo Emerson

D. Sims was a kind and gentle man, full of humor, always with a story to tell. I knew him well and liked him. He was one of the first oncologists in our city and had built a fine practice. He was a Christian doctor who felt a responsibility toward the poor. One day an uninsured young man came to him with cancer. There was real hope that this young man might be cured of his cancer with appropriate therapy, but he had no medical insurance. It is not clear why Dr. Sims agreed to manage this young man's care, but the assumption was that his motives were purely charitable. The man received his therapy, but was not cured and eventually died of his disease.

About a year later Dr. Sims lost a lawsuit for his part in the young man's death. The claim was made, and the jury agreed, that Dr. Sims had chosen substandard chemotherapy because he could get that medicine more cheaply than the standard therapy and thus would lose less money in his patient's care. Dr. Sims lost his appeal and forfeited his home and retirement income. He himself died soon after the appeal from pancreatic cancer, leaving his wife alone in a small apartment. If the jury was correct in their verdict, Dr. Sims had good intentions and a kind heart, both rendered ineffective by a problem in character. Character is a complicated issue.

—A Christian Doctor

In the 1990s, while the debate raged in politics about whether character is an essential component of leadership, corporate scandals were brewing that would later erupt in the business world and settle the issue, at least

The temptation to step across moral boundary lines is something that tests every doctor's character.

for this generation. Enron, Global Crossing, and Tyco, just to name a few of those that got caught, taught us that choosing leaders without character, no matter how competent, is a costly venture. Sadly, politics and business are not the only arenas where character failure can be catastrophic.

In its seventy-fifth anniversary issue, *Medical Economics* magazine noted several doctors who arguably failed the test of character. Orthopedist John Nork admitted in court that for nine years he made a practice of "performing surgery and performing it badly," just for the cash. Everyone complains about reimbursement problems, but another doctor, cardiologist Richard Kones, collected $1.3 million in bogus reimbursement claims from Medicare, Medicaid, workman's compensation, Social Security, and six insurance companies before pleading guilty to first-degree larceny.

And, if you're looking for the record number of malpractice claims, plastic surgeon Richard Dombroff could well hold the dishonor at two hundred twelve. He built a mini-empire based on the concept of same-day cosmetic surgery at his "Personal Best" center in Manhattan. At its peak, Dombroff's practice performed five thousand operations a year, generating a gross profit of about $5 million. His assembly-line approach to nose jobs, tummy tucks, and breast implants made Dombroff a rich man–temporarily–but at the expense of his patients. Eventually, Dombroff pleaded guilty to fraud for billing for reconstructive rather than cosmetic surgery. All but one of the malpractice claims against him had to be settled in a bankruptcy court.

Although men and women like these are the exceptions rather than the rule, the temptation to step across moral boundary lines is something that tests every doctor's character. They remind us that character is important and that there is something desperately wrong in the hearts of men and women.

THE CHARACTER COLLISION

While the legal system has shined its light on this "dark side of medicine," there are plenty of other ethical situations unbounded by law or ethical consensus. Relativistic thinking has corroded the moral anchor of medicine. "Can we?" is rapidly replacing "Should we?" The fact is, it's legal to do the wrong thing in many situations. Just looking at physician-assisted suicide and the current ethical quandaries in genetics demands that Christians consider seriously how they will respond when money, major social pressures, and the natural demands of medical practice collide with their convictions.

Sad but true, while medical science is looking for answers, the church is stuttering. Once dominant in healthcare, the church has largely disengaged. And what's more tragic, many Christian physicians have run for cover or become morally camouflaged. Often in the doctor's lounge, it's hard to tell many Christian doctors from non-Christian doctors. They tend to use the same inappropriate language, tell the same off-color jokes, entertain themselves with the same questionable movies and TV, treat their coworkers with the same lack of dignity, and love their families only when it's convenient. They tend to drive with the same ferociousness toward the same ends as non-Christians—power, position, and possessions. Increasingly, the only difference between Christians and their non-Christian colleagues is where they go after rounds on Sunday morning. These aren't issues settled by improving medical competence or taking ethical decision-making courses. In many cases the only thing holding back a moral cave-in is the character of the doctor. As co-author of "The Saline Solution," Walt Larimore says, "Character without competence is sentimental. But competence without character is scary." Certainly it is scary for patients, scary for medicine, but also scary for the doctor.

In the rush to provide "character curriculum" to fill the moral vacuum of turn-of-the-century America, healthcare has not been overlooked. In recent years, many medical organizations, including the American Board of Internal Medicine (ABIM), Association of American Medical Colleges (AAMC), and the American Medical Association (AMA), have developed initiatives to strengthen medical professionalism and ethics. In a recent book, the author's list of virtues includes "a deep capacity for compassion, truthfulness, trustworthiness, courage, humility, and a consistent inclination to act justly."

Over ten years ago Dr. Edmund Pellegrino, founder of The Center for Clinical Bioethics and now Professor Emeritus of Medicine and Medical Ethics at Georgetown University, warned of the essential need for character development in physicians. "In addition to cognitive and behavioral skills, some attention must be paid to the affective component of clinical ethics–that is to say, to the kind of person the physician should be as well as the kind of decisions he or she should make," Pellegrino wrote. "In short, ethics requires that the physician be a person who can be expected to habitually act in the patient's interests when no one is watching."[1]

Why is character essential for the doctor? Because great gifts, great skill, great learning, must be governed by great virtue. Again, Dr. Pellegrino wrote, "All medical ethics finally rest on the physician's moral character. In those moments of clinical decision, when no one is watching, the physician's character is the patient's last safeguard."[2]

In the place of incredible vulnerability, the patient needs to know that his or her doctor practices good medicine, and can be trusted to have the

"Character without competence is sentimental. But competence without character is scary." –Walt Larimore

Character is the inner compass that sets our course when the road signs of life don't give clear directions.

patient's best interest at heart. Without character, the great skills and learning of the physician make him or her into a curse, not a blessing, to society.

The word *character* comes from a Greek word meaning to engrave. Different symbols in the alphabet came to be called characters; that is, they each have a distinctive look given by the engraver so they can be told apart. So, character came to mean the distinctive marks or the combination of traits and qualities distinguishing the individual nature of a thing or person. The word's origin gives us a graphic illustration of what character represents in a person. Our character is that which distinguishes us – sets us apart. It's that which is engraved in "granite" on our hearts – what we can be counted on to be like without fail. Or as Dr. Pellegrino suggests, "who we are when no one is watching." Character is the inner compass that sets our course when the road signs of life don't give clear directions.

THE DEVELOPMENT OF CHRISTIAN CHARACTER

Though the Bible never uses this particular Greek word, the formation of character, the distinctive internal qualities God wants a person to possess, is one of the central themes of the New Testament. When Jesus instructs his disciples to go and make disciples, he's commanding them to do more than preach a gospel of forgiveness. He's challenging them to offer a new life – a life of companionship with God, a friendship that will transform people's lives from the inside out, making them into new people. To say it another way, we don't need a plastic surgeon; we need a cardiologist. We don't need a new look; we need a new heart.

God is not only interested in changing and perfecting our behavior–how we look–he is interested in changing who we are, so that our "distinguishing marks" look like Jesus. Not only is a disciple one who follows and learns, but one who wants to become like his or her master. Jesus said, "A disciple is not above his teacher, but everyone who is perfectly trained will be like his teacher" (Luke 6:40, NKJV).

Don't misunderstand. Discipleship is not some industrial-strength version of the Christian life. It is the street-level enterprise of every member of God's kingdom. And it should be the aim of every doctor who names the name of Jesus as Savior, to bring the character of Jesus into his or her practice. This is evident in the pages of the New Testament. Before your attending sought to mold you into a doctor, God determined to conform your character to the likeness of Jesus: "For those God foreknew he also predestined to be conformed to the likeness of his Son, that he might be the firstborn among many brothers" (Rom. 8:29).

It is a distinct possibility that the shape of your practice might look just like any worldly doctor's unless your character is reshaped and your mind is renewed in the knowledge of Jesus: "Do not conform any longer to the pattern of this world, but be transformed by the renewing of your mind. Then you will be able to test and approve what God's will is – his good, pleasing and perfect will" (Rom. 12:2).

As intellectually superior as you may be, you still need to mature spiritually and you still need correction from God's Word: "We proclaim him, admonishing and teaching everyone with all wisdom, so that we may present everyone perfect in Christ" (Col. 1:28). "My dear children, for whom I am again in the pains of childbirth until Christ is formed in you" (Gal. 4:19).

Developing godly character is a lifelong process of claiming and experiencing the life that is already ours in abundance in Jesus. Real change is not only possible, it is the natural outcome of continually choosing to follow Jesus and be like our master:

> His divine power has given us everything we need for life and godliness through our knowledge of him who called us by his own glory and goodness. Through these he has given us his very great and precious promises, so that through them you may participate in the divine nature and escape the corruption in the world caused by evil desires. For this very reason, make every effort to add to your faith goodness; and to goodness, knowledge; and to knowledge, self-control; and to self-control, perseverance; and to perseverance, godliness; and to godliness, brotherly kindness; and to brotherly kindness, love. For if you possess these qualities in increasing measure, they will keep you from being ineffective and unproductive in your knowledge of our Lord Jesus Christ. But if anyone does not have them, he is nearsighted and blind, and has forgotten that he has been cleansed from his past sins (2 Pet. 1:3-9).

Perhaps the clearest contrast in character and the clearest description of our need to change is found in Galatians 5 where Paul makes the comparison between the person we are naturally and the person we can be as a result of the Spirit's work:

> So I say, live by the Spirit, and you will not gratify the desires of the sinful nature. For the sinful nature desires what is contrary to the Spirit and the Spirit what is contrary to the sinful nature. They are in conflict with each other, so that you do not do what you want. But if you are led by the Spirit, you are not under law. The acts of the sinful nature are obvious: sexual immorality, impurity

Developing godly character is a lifelong process of claiming and experiencing the life that is already ours in abundance in Jesus.

and debauchery; idolatry and witchcraft; hatred, discord, jealousy, fits of rage, selfish ambition, dissensions, factions and envy; drunkenness, orgies, and the like. I warn you, as I did before, that those who live like this will not inherit the kingdom of God. But the fruit of the Spirit is love, joy, peace, patience, kindness, goodness, faithfulness, gentleness and self-control. Against such things there is no law. Those who belong to Christ Jesus have crucified the sinful nature with its passions and desires. Since we live by the Spirit, let us keep in step with the Spirit (Gal. 5:16-25).

This passage gives us hope that no matter how old we are, or how hardened our character has become, there is the possibility of positive character development. It is by no means, however, automatic for a Christian. As Paul implies, transformation is the Spirit's work, but elsewhere he makes it clear that our cooperation is involved.

Our cooperation is most valuable in the two areas of shaping our environment and choosing our focus. As children, it is difficult to control our environment and the shaping influences on our lives that we are immersed in. But, as adults, we select and even shape our own environment in many ways.

Doctors who choose to follow Jesus are still faced with the powerful pressure of a culture that pushes them away from God and toward the behaviors and values of the person they used to be. If it's not immorality, impurity and debauchery, it is pride that produces hatred, discord, jealousy, or greed that leads to selfish ambition and envy. At the end of this path is a hollowness that drives us to addictions and anything that will soothe the pain of emptiness.

Historically, Christians have tried to escape this path by isolating themselves in solitary settings or enclaves. Sometimes, when Christians are weaker than the environment, removing themselves from that environment is essential—as when doctors who are addicted to pornography need to avoid being alone in hotel rooms with cable television. But as Christians have consistently discovered, it is easier to get the Christian out of the world than it is to get the world out of the Christian. Isolation from bad influences is not the ultimate answer to our character weaknesses.

In Colossians, Paul reminds us that real change isn't a product of environment, but a product of our focus within that environment. While living in the midst of earthly temptations and professional tensions, change comes from focusing on Jesus and the heavenly realities of who he has transformed me to be: "Since, then, you have been raised with Christ, set your hearts on things above, where Christ is seated at the right hand of God. Set your minds on things above, not on earthly things (Col. 3:1-2).

This is not some legalistic duty, but the privilege of Jesus' followers, which brings hope for genuine change over time in our character—no matter how hardened the shape of our hearts may be, or the way we were raised, or the poor choices we made in the past. Paul continues:

> Put to death, therefore, whatever belongs to your earthly nature: sexual immorality, impurity, lust, evil desires and greed, which is idolatry. Because of these, the wrath of God is coming. You used to walk in these ways, in the life you once lived. But now you must rid yourselves of all such things as these: anger, rage, malice, slander, and filthy language from your lips. Do not lie to one another (Col. 3:5-9).

The Bible ought to sit next to every physician's PDR and be consulted at least as frequently.

These outward changes, the result of focusing on Christ, are made possible because he is doing something deep inside us. Paul continues, "...since you have taken off your old self with its practices and have put on the new self, which is being renewed in knowledge in the image of its Creator" (Col. 3:9-10).

Our intake of God's Word obviously plays an important role in this transformation. It is our new source of truth and reality. It gives a solid way to evaluate the environment we live in—every circumstance and situation we face. As we focus on Christ and let him speak to us through his Word, the Spirit reshapes our hearts so that his thoughts and character take up residence there. That's why Paul reminds us to, "Let the word of Christ dwell in you richly as you teach and admonish one another with all wisdom, and as you sing psalms, hymns and spiritual songs with gratitude in your hearts to God" (Col. 3:16).

The Bible ought to sit next to every physician's PDR and be consulted at least as frequently. The goal is not to know just the facts of God's word, any more than it would be for a doctor to memorize the PDR just to know medications. To be worthwhile, the information must be used to heal, in this case, our own lives.

Character development is not something one does in isolation. The reason other individuals have such a shaping influence on our lives, positive and negative, is that God created us to be social beings. And just as some people can lead us astray, others can lead us to the truth. God's desire is that, no matter how difficult the flow of culture and pressure from the people we work with, we have a group of fellow followers of Jesus to help us stay on track. We need Jesus, but we need each other also, to remind us of the reality of our identity in Christ, the actuality of our relationship with Jesus, and credibility of God's Word.

"Non-discipleship costs abiding peace, a life penetrated throughout by love, faith that sees everything in the light of God's overriding governance for good, hopefulness that stands firm in the most discouraging of circumstances, power to do what is right and withstand the forces of evil."
—Dallas Willard

The sad fact is this: Christians who isolate themselves from other followers of Jesus almost always succumb to the shaping pressure of the culture. In the culture of medicine, that is a frightening prospect. Not only will patients' individual welfare be threatened, but Christians will fail to bring any shaping influence on the culture itself.

The Real Tragedy

The greatest threat in a lack of character is to the doctor himself or herself. Discipleship sometimes demands an exacting price and the journey to becoming like Jesus is at times a costly trek. But Christian doctors should also count the cost of non-discipleship—the cost of choosing not to follow Jesus. In his book *The Spirit of the Disciplines*, Dallas Willard states, "Non-discipleship costs abiding peace, a life penetrated throughout by love, faith that sees everything in the light of God's overriding governance for good, hopefulness that stands firm in the most discouraging of circumstances, power to do what is right and withstand the forces of evil. In short, it costs exactly that abundance of life Jesus said he came to bring (John10:10)."[3]

To fail your patients is dreadful. To fail your calling is tragic. To fail to live up to your true identity as a child of God—to be conformed to Christ's character—is to miss life itself.

Action Plan

So how do we go about it? First, how do we evaluate the character that we demonstrate to others? Then, how do we remold the areas of our lives that do not fit the character of Christ?

One of the things that we need to do as we look at this question of character is to evaluate ourselves. Do we measure up to God's standards? Only God knows, and though we may prefer to live comfortably with ourselves not knowing, it is better that we understand ourselves. Perhaps then we can work out our salvation as Paul asks us to.

When we look at the big picture and ask why God keeps us on this earth rather than sending us ahead to a better place, there seem to be only two reasons: one is to bring others to him; the other is to give us the time and opportunity to become more like Christ. If we seek to accomplish the latter, we need to understand our character so that we can work with God in areas where we are weak.

Let's take a quiz. Review the following situations and decide how you would respond. Make a list of the character qualities that compete in your decision making and rate your personal score in those qualities from 1-4, with 4 being the highest in relation to each case. For example, in the first situation, 1 might be a desire to protect yourself and 4 might be complete truthfulness.

1. You gave a patient a medicine to which she is allergic. The allergy note was in your record, but you failed to review it. The patient became quite ill and spent three days in the hospital recovering. She is not aware of the connection between her illness and the medicine you gave. When the patient returns to your office after the hospital stay, she asks, "Doctor, do you know what caused me to be so sick?"

2. Your patient calls with a painful tooth or a terrible rash. Both could wait until the next day, but this patient has an aggravating personality. He insists on taking care of it today in spite of your full schedule and early plans at home.

3. A patient you have treated for years through many serious difficulties comes to you with a new problem that you can handle well, but her best friend gave her the name of one of your competitors in town who advertises his skill with the illness she now has. She asks if you would send a copy of her records to that doctor to see how he would handle it.

4. You are an hour behind in your office day. You walk into a room where you cringe because you know the patient is incredibly verbose, with many social problems unrelated to the physical problem for which she came to you. There are tears in her eyes. "Doctor," she says, "so much has gone wrong since I was here last. I've made a list so I wouldn't forget anything."

5. Your spouse calls in the middle of a very busy day to say that your son's principal has called. Your son has been suspended for having marijuana in his locker. Many patients are waiting to be seen.

6. You ask an employee to help a patient to her car because she is light-headed and you are afraid she will fall. Your employee says, "I'm about to go on my lunch break. You will have to find someone else."

7. You have been up all night in the emergency room or with a sick spouse. The person who is helping you move patients to examining rooms today is distracted by her new engagement ring and is constantly chatting with fellow employees while your rooms are slow to fill.

Your spouse has been distant lately. A very nice colleague to whom you are attracted suggests that you have lunch together.

Take the picture of your own character and place it next to a character portrait of Jesus Christ. If you are satisfied, you either have come very close to God's plan for character in your life, or you are so far from it that you don't really understand the character of Christ.

8. The time has come to decide how much to raise your patient fees this year.

9. You are discussing how to deal with uninsured patients with your associates.

10. Your spouse has been distracted by work for six months and very distant in spite of your protests. A very nice colleague to whom you are attracted suggests that you have lunch together.

11. You casually clicked upon a pornographic e-mail last week and were stimulated by the pictures. You are now in a hotel room and flipping through the movie channels where one option is erotic movies.

12. You have a choice tonight between attending your regular small group Bible study or using tickets to see your favorite professional team play.

13. You promised your partners that you would stay with the group for at least three more years when they made their plans for office space. A new job opportunity has offered you a 50 percent increase if you come this year.

14. You have a choice between two procedures. Both are equally efficacious for the problem. One remunerates you much more than the other. They both are well covered by insurance.

How did you do? Your character evaluation does not come with right or wrong answers, for there may be many ways to work out each situation. The evaluation of your character comes when you recognize the places you struggle—or fail to struggle within each situation.

The next step is to take the picture of your own character and place it next to a character portrait of Jesus Christ. If you are satisfied, you either have come very close to God's plan for character in your life, or you are so far from it that you don't really understand the character of Christ.

Use the following list to help you make your comparison:

• Never tell a lie, even if you die (Prov. 12:19).
• Welcome every struggle as a chance to lean on God and persevere (Heb. 10:36-38).
• We must obey God rather than men (Acts 5:29).

◆See kindness as an accomplishment greater than any urgent goals (Eph. 4:32).

◆In humility count others better than yourselves (Phil. 2:4-8).

◆Resist the devil and he will flee from you. Come near to God and he will come near to you (James 4:7-8).

◆Can you take instruction well? (Prov. 19:20).

◆Do you have a problem with laziness? (Prov. 19:15; Prov. 18:9).

◆How is your pride? (Prov. 16:5; Prov. 18:2).

◆Do you live a contented life? (Phil. 4:11-13).

◆How is your patience? (Prov. 25:15).

◆Can you control your anger? (Prov. 27:4).

"God has not called me to be successful. He has called me to be faithful."
—Mother Teresa

START TO CHANGE:

After comparing your life to the list above, how do you measure up? If you are not satisfied, the following will help guide your change. Keep in mind that character comes not from indoctrination but from immersion.

NINE ACTIONS TO CONSIDER

1. Be certain that you have been immersed in God's Spirit through a saving relationship with Jesus Christ.

2. Make the commitment to follow Christ as Lord of you life, in spite of other attractions.

3. List the attractions that have drawn you away from the Lordship of Christ, lay them at the foot of the cross and do not pick them up again.

4. Study God's Word faithfully daily and ask each day, "How does this Word affect my walk today?" Think of one practical application for each day and commit to it.

5. Establish yourself in a small group of Christians for discussion, accountability, and prayer. Meet on a regular basis.

6. For difficult character flaws, set up pastoral counseling sessions.

7. Read biographies of great men and women who demonstrated great character. Identify those character traits that you desire and hold up that man or woman as a hero to follow in those traits (examples might include Teddy Roosevelt, Abraham Lincoln, George Washington, John Adams, Oswald Chambers, Jim Elliot, Dietrich Bonhoeffer, Martin Luther, Helen Keller, Mother Teresa, Robert E. Lee, Booker T. Washington, Mahatma Gandhi).

8. Each day give all of your life, relationships, possessions, family members, dreams, and sins to God in prayer.

9. Listen for God's direction as you pray.

PRAYER

Dear Father,
I am not who I wish to be. Take out of my life those flaws that keep me from being
good in your eyes. Place within me the character I need to live out the mission
that you created me to accomplish. Let others see Jesus in me.

—Amen

NOTES:

1. Pellegrino, E,D, Siegler, M., Singer, P.A. "Teaching clinical ethics." *Journal of Clinical Ethics* 1990; 1:175–180.
2. Ibid.
3. Dallas Willard, *The Spirit of the Disciplines*, San Francisco: HarperSanFrancisco, 1988, p. 263.

CHAPTER 4

Competence

"Whatever your task, work heartily, as serving the Lord and not men, knowing that from the Lord you will receive the inheritance as your reward; you are serving the Lord Christ" (Col. 3:23-24, RSV).

*H*alf way across the Pacific Ocean on a night flight to Thailand (and on my way to teach at the biennial CMDA-CMDE [Continuing Medical & Dental Education] conference), I heard the flight attendant urgently call for a doctor aboard the plane. Eight hours earlier I had boarded the flight, tired but hoping to have several hours of protected time to review my teaching notes for the next two weeks. And now...this call.

Knowing that nothing happens outside the Lord's plans, and sensing that there might be a way to assist in mid-air, I bounded up from my economy seat and quickly located the panicked flight attendant with a male passenger who had just had a seizure. Several other doctors had also responded to the call, but when I volunteered that I was a neurologist, the others deferred.

Fortunately, the passenger's wife was accompanying him on the flight and could provide useful information about his epilepsy; on the other hand, her husband (my patient) resisted my examination and inquiries. From her, I first took a neurological history and then quickly ran through my list: Precipitating events? Medication use? Compliance and therapeutic levels? Last dose? Recent changes? Last food or drink? Concurrent medical problems? I performed a focused physical exam as best could be done in that cramped setting – then pondered the plan of action.

With hours to go before reaching any airfield, the question was what to do at 30,000 feet up in the air. What were the risks and benefits of diverting from our flight pattern, versus staying the course and seeking medical care on arrival in Taipei five hours away?

Does it matter to God whether Christian doctors are excellent doctors and good witnesses, rather than just fair doctors and good witnesses?

After a quiet prayer and quick reflection from my experience with other similar patients, I chose to stay the course and seek further assistance when we landed as scheduled. Over the rest of the flight I closely monitored my patient. I was relieved that his post-ictal period was brief and that he eventually regained his orientation and faculties. The Lord's guidance, coupled with my years of neurology expertise, helped make a decision which was in the best interests of the patient, which benefited other passengers, and which carried credibility and authority.

When I arrived in Thailand for the CMDA-CMDE conference, a colleague approached me with a challenging consultation: our keynote speaker (a surgeon) was said "not to be himself." According to his wife, he had recently been unable to perform double-digit multiplication in his head, and normally spry in step, he had occasionally tripped on sidewalk curbs. The patient himself downplayed these observations, attributing them to jet lag, weariness as a reluctant tourist at the side of his energetic wife, and long hours in the operating room just before the journey to Thailand. He insisted he was fine and would soon be back to his usual ways. My careful history and detailed review of systems revealed no clues. His physical and mental exams were entirely normal – except for the last thing on a neurological exam: plantar reflexes. He had one up-going toe. Consistently. That sign changed the whole picture, and I explained my finding and my concern to him and his wife.

As a doctor, he had brushed aside all concerns prior to this. Now we were talking about something serious, something possibly intracranial. Within a matter of hours, we had located a Thai neuroradiologist at a local hospital, and the diagnosis was confirmed: bilateral subdural hematomas, dating to a slow leak from minor (and historically forgotten) occipital head trauma months before. Over time the patient had gradually compensated until the bleeding volume could no longer be accommodated by the intracranial space. The patient went immediately to the local Thai operating room. Within a week, we had our keynote speaker back, grinning and sporting a baseball cap over his shaved head and the sutured areas where the neurosurgeon had been at work to drain the subdurals and relieve the intracranial pressure. Clinical excellence and team work made all the difference.

–Clydette Powell, M.D.

WHAT IS COMPETENCE (OR EXCELLENCE) IN MEDICINE AND DENTISTRY?

If excellence is defined as being "exceptionally good of its kind," does such a virtue matter to God? Does it matter to God whether Christian doctors are excellent doctors and good witnesses, rather than just fair doctors and good witnesses?

It certainly does. The Bible abounds with examples of excellence that served the Lord's purposes. Jesus himself was the paragon of excellence in medical practice, manifesting all the qualities to which we aspire as health-care practitioners. He readily saw into the body, heart, and mind of all those who sought him. He understood the physical and spiritual reasons for health and illness. He took time for people, treating them as individuals in need of health and healing. He was a skilled craftsman at what he did. His work as a Master Physician was renowned, and people sought after him.

As we seek to be like our Lord in other ways, we should seek to serve our patients with competent medical care. How do we define such competence? Competence requires both knowledge and performance. The foundation of medical competence is knowledge, and this knowledge is more than just textbook learning or being chief resident. The word *know* in Hebrew implies a depth of understanding, and implies thoroughness and completeness derived by intimate contact with a subject or person. Knowledge is coupled with skillfulness or craftsmanship. Such workmanship is represented by the ability to take something and fashion it into something of great worth.

For example, when the Lord, through Moses, commissioned builders for his temple, he wanted things worked by a skilled craftsmen–see Ex. 26:31. While Moses was up on Mount Sinai getting the Ten Commandments, the Lord indicated that he wanted skilled craftsmen, and he helped them get the work done by filling them with the Holy Spirit.

Excellence in scientific medicine exemplifies the highest and finest quality in diagnosing, treating, and preventing disease in the body and mind. Such excellence may be evident within an individual patient consultation or within a public health intervention for a whole community of people. It may be demonstrated within a classroom, a court room, a board room, a research laboratory, or under a mango tree. The excellent practitioner of medicine may be an individual clinician in practice, an academician at a university medical school, a research scientist, public health specialist, a missionary physician, or a physician executive in a management setting.

Excellence in the practice of medicine may lead Christians to assume positions of influence in healthcare and health policy:

♦Francis Collins, a physician-geneticist, holds the reins of leadership as Director of the National Human Genome Research Institute at the National Institutes of Health. The Human Genome Project, which is mapping and sequencing the entire human DNA, is regarded by some as the most significant scientific research undertaken in our time.

Excellence in the practice of medicine may lead Christians to assume positions of influence in healthcare and health policy.

Where do you stand in your own desire for excellence in your corner of God's world?

♦Edmund Pellegrino, Professor Emeritus of Medicine and Medical Ethics at Georgetown University School of Medicine in Washington, D.C., debates many within the nation's capital and beyond about the sanctity of life as well as end-of-life decisions coming from our courts of law.

♦Paul and Margaret Brand, both physicians, served many years on the mission field, while pioneering in the care of leprosy patients and those afflicted with eye disease.

♦Helen Roseveare, a physician in the medical missions field, dedicated a lifetime of excellence in medicine to poor communities in rural Zaire (present-day Democratic Republic of the Congo). Moreover, she multiplied her talents by establishing a training center in Zaire, by teaching local and foreign healthcare providers, and by authoring books to inspire others to service and excellence in medicine.

♦Jacob Kumaresan, an Indian infectious disease specialist, led the STOP TB Secretariat for the World Health Organization and now serves as the Executive Director for the International Trachoma Institute. With his leadership he is having a kingdom impact on those suffering from tuberculosis and eye disease in the developing world.

♦Elaine Eng, an Asian-American psychiatrist, ministers locally through her practice in New York and also globally to missionaries serving in remote places. Trained as an obstetrician-gynecologist, Elaine had to switch specialties when her eyesight deteriorated to legal blindness due to retinitis pigmentosa while a surgical resident and young mother.

Elaine turned that physical adversity into something beautiful for the Lord. Unable to see her patients, she learned to listen to the heart better than any cardiologist. She became fully adept at making mental notes of what her patients told her – and remembering what sighted doctors would need recorded in charts and dictated notes for recall.

To large audiences, Elaine speaks authoritatively, with literature references, memorized, on topics of psychiatric disorders. Undistracted visually, her listening skills are finely tuned, functioning as excellent receptors for making a diagnosis and offering wise, scripturally–based counsel.

With her quiet and unrushed demeanor, she listens intently, and then lifts and redirects the hurting soul to Christ, using her excellence in psychiatry to make the diagnosis and offer the treatment.

One person at a time, Elaine ministers to those who work in remote and challenging settings. Her medical excellence is fully applied to building and re-equipping the Lord's laborers in the field.

Where do you stand in your own desire for excellence in your corner of God's world? Do you consider yourself a skilled craftsman? Are you as good a doctor as you have ever been? Have you allowed your knowledge and technical skills to lapse with time because other areas of your life seem to be more important? Is it really that important to practice excellence when we barely have enough time to be adequate?

WHY SHOULD WE AIM TO EXCEL IN OUR WORK?

Excellence takes work. Excellence can take time away from other priorities like family, fun, and worship. Should we really sacrifice important life at home in order to be better at work, realizing we spend too much time at work anyway? The question of time at home is an important one that will be addressed elsewhere, but I believe God wants us to find the means to be *excellent* in each of the tasks he gives us to do.

First of all, **we are designed for excellence** by the Master Craftsman. We are designed to be "...God's workmanship, created in Christ Jesus to do good works, which God prepared in advance for us to do" (Eph. 2: 10). In addition, God expects us to continue to grow, just as Peter wrote in his second letter to a wide circle of early Christians: "But grow in the grace and knowledge of our Lord and Savior Jesus Christ. To him be glory both now and forever!" (2 Pet. 3:18).

Secondly, in view of these principles, **we are commanded to be excellent**, regardless of our setting and niche within medicine. We are exhorted to do with all our might whatever our hands find to do (Eccl. 9:10). We are commanded in the New Testament: "Whatever you do, work at it with all your heart, as working for the Lord, not for men, since you know that you will receive an inheritance from the Lord as a reward. It is the Lord Christ you are serving" (Col. 3: 23).

In other words, there is no back-seat, optional job, if we are obedient and use all that the Lord has given us. We are instructed to keep our minds set on the highest standards. In his letter to the Philippians, Paul reminds us: "Finally brothers, whatever is true, whatever is noble, whatever is right, whatever is pure, whatever is lovely, whatever is admirable—if anything is excellent or praiseworthy—think about such things" (Phil. 4:8).

We are to hold fast to certain core values and Christlike practices, focusing our minds on what is the best.

God wants us to find the means to be excellent in each of the tasks he gives us to do.

*The quality
of our work
and service is
more than
just a part
of our
professional
persona;
it is an
important
part of
our witness
for Christ.*

Thirdly, we need to recognize that **it is not our efforts, but the Lord's blessing, that endows our work with value**. "May the favor of the Lord our God rest upon us; establish the work of our hands for us – yes, establish the work of our hands" (Ps. 90:17). The Holy Spirit makes that difference in the quality of our work. The infilling of the Holy Spirit distinguishes us from other skilled workers. Moses records such an infilling for excellence in the verses surrounding Ex. 31:3 : "...I have filled him [Bezalel] with the Spirit of God, with skill, ability and knowledge in all kinds of crafts."

A fourth consideration is that **excellence confers the power of influence**. People will be inclined to listen to us because of our competence and excellence. Joseph, Esther, and Daniel all catapulted to levels of influence because of their excellence. Nehemiah rose to a position of influence as cupbearer to the king, a most trusted position.

"Do you see a man skilled in his work?" Solomon wrote. "He will serve before kings; he will not serve before obscure men" (Prov. 22:29). As King, David shepherded his people with "integrity of heart; with skillful hands he led them" (Ps. 78:72).

We need to seek grace to work hard and well at whatever the Lord gives us, because the quality of our work and service is more than just a part of our professional persona; it is an important part of our witness for Christ. It is important to try to deliver more than simply the expected service, and always to give that service our very best attempts. If others see substandard work, they may associate this with being a Christian and thus discredit our faith and effective witness. People won't be able to see beyond our mediocrity.

On the other hand, if we show ourselves to be excellent, even though others might disagree or even attack us, we will have won their respect. We will be credible; this is our platform on which to speak and to have influence for Christ, the light of the world. Just as light does not exist to demonstrate its own beauty, excellence exists to point the way to something else on which our eyes should be fixed. It best serves when it is a steady and consistent light, shining without flickering and having enough wattage to reveal what it is meant to show.

In our own work, excellence is a light shining to reveal Christ to others. Our consistent witness to them through competency in our practice helps to direct the vision of others away from ourselves and to the One whose Name is above all names. People will notice our excellence. People will listen to our message. People will be drawn closer to our Lord.

Finally, **excellent medical and dental care improves the lives of the suffering people whom God loves**. Jesus did not heal the sick only to get them to heaven. Jesus healed the sick because he loved them; they were his children suffering in a broken world. Love does not reach out with leftovers. Love reaches out with the best we have to those we love and who need us. Half-hearted excellence in medical and dental care suggests half-hearted love and thereby fails to demonstrate the presence of Christ to those who are suffering and whom we serve.

WHAT CAN WE DO TO PRACTICE EXCELLENCE?

What can we do, and who can we be, to keep that light shining brightly, to build the kingdom, and to preserve the high quality of service to which we are called? How are we to distinguish ourselves as distinctly Christian – and excellent – in this twenty-first century? How are we to find the way through landmines of medical error and patient safety issues? How can our light shine clearly and competently in this ever-evolving world of medical and public health challenges? How can we put in place what the Lord requires of us as his ambassadors here on earth? Let me propose some steps that can guide you on the path to excellence, for his purposes and his kingdom here on earth:

How can we put in place what the Lord requires of us as his ambassadors here on earth?

1. Begin and end all your work with prayer. Surround it and instill it into your desire to do God's will on earth. Jesus did the same. Scripture often reports Jesus being in prayer. His very life ended with the satisfaction of having been obedient to the end.

2. Have an unquenchable thirst for learning. The wonders of God's creation are available to us when we show interest and make the effort to understand what he has revealed through scientific discovery. So, delight in learning. Establish a lifelong learning plan. Make it part of your lifestyle; pursue knowledge. Remember that being able to formulate questions may be more important than being able to answer them. Keep your learning style active rather than passive. Try different forms of learning – journals, conferences, tapes and CDs, online learning – and vary them. It will at times require perseverance, discipline, and doggedness, especially when other demands crowd in. Set reasonable goals with target dates. Consider setting aside time to master a focused topic.

3. Read. This is one easy way to continue to learn. Reading with a specific goal or a question in mind is easier, with the result that the educational points are more likely to stick. Reflect as you read. Confucius said, "Reading without thinking is null and void, whereas thinking without

"Reading without thinking is null and void, whereas thinking without reading is critical and full of risk."
—Confucius

reading is critical and full of risk." Yet with the plethora of medical journals and "throw-away" publications, how can we choose the best among many to read? Look for recognized authors in their field as well as relevance to your own interests. Next, skim the methodology. Were these the results of a randomized controlled trial, a case-control study, or an isolated case report? What is the scientific validity of the article? In the 1990's the *Journal of the American Medical Association* launched a series on "Reading the Medical Literature," a timeless guide for the discerning and busy reader.

4. Express yourself in writing and public speaking. Writing case reports, review articles, original research, and even news briefs keeps you fresh and responsible to colleagues, who will critique your public presentations. Writing and speaking require critical and analytical thinking. Moreover, writing and speaking help improve your abilities to communicate on paper and in person. Being able to get ideas across is invaluable in patient care. Participate on committees that can provide you with visibility and may lead to opportunities to be of influence as a Christian in your field.

5. Teach others. Teaching is a proven stimulus to excellence. Young medical students and residents with inquiring minds will help you to revisit the basics, as well as stay up-to-date. As Alfred North Whitehead said, "Knowledge does not keep any better than fish." Teaching will make you organize your knowledge for presentation and will be the natural forum for feedback about your strengths or inadequacies. Moreover, it is the guarantee to keep your "intellectual epiphyses" from closing!

6. Find a mentor. Surround yourself with those who can teach you. Find someone who takes an interest in you. Consider writing papers with someone. Jesus was the ideal mentor to his disciples. Although we do not have earthly mentors quite like Jesus, look for those mentors who manifest Christlike qualities, as they can have a major influence in your life and practice. Mentors can provide guidance on career choices or changes, can offer perspective on patient treatment options, and can be there for support when you face dilemmas in patient care.

7. Become and remain credentialed. Although credentials do not represent the entire picture of excellence in craftsmanship, they testify that we meet widely recognized standards and are thereby qualified to practice in our field. They do not guarantee, however, that the knowledge is practiced, since knowledge does not equate with skill.

If you are not yet board certified in your practice area, begin the process to prepare for those exams. If you are already board certified, keep up your knowledge and re-certify when indicated by your board. Credentials carry much influence; in some settings board certification is required for admitting privileges within hospitals, managed care plans, and in some instances to hold positions of responsibility and influence. The apostle Paul recognized the weight of credentials when he presented his own to both the Philippians (Phil. 3:5) and the Corinthians (2 Cor. 11: 22-33). He spoke of his training and his excellence. He applied those credentials effectively in communicating with people of different cultures and backgrounds: the Jewish Christians (Acts 15), the Greek philosophers (Acts 17), local churches, and Roman rulers. From the Old Testament, we see that Solomon's wisdom was a gift of God and, in a sense, his credential for being king of all Israel. It gained him deep respect from the people he served.

Your efforts to understand other cultures will provide you an invaluable window on the world.

8. Get to know other cultures. Be a kind of medical anthropologist. Your efforts to understand other cultures will provide you an invaluable window on the world. Try to grasp how others define illness or health, what approaches they use to treat diseases, and what non-medical factors contribute to the health problems in their community. Connect with colleagues outside your geographical area of practice.

I learned from my Cambodian colleagues all that I know about dengue hemorrhagic fever in children; this was hands-on knowledge which never could have been extracted from a textbook. Moreover, by studying the Khmer language, I came to discover cultural attitudes about epilepsy, about village management of measles, about death and dying, and about Cambodian redistributive justice. By working in Zaire, I developed an understanding of the role of village "witch doctors" and how they could create new problems for us, thwart our well-reasoned medical interventions, or be potential links in the early identification of illness.

—Clydette Powell M.D.

Cultural lessons such as these can teach us why some people groups may refuse immunization or have unusual sexual practices, or why some diseases such as AIDS and TB carry significant stigmas. The study of people provides clues to effective and excellent healthcare service. Learn from these patients and populations. You may want to consider short-term missions to accomplish this.

Healing occurs when excellence and love are poured out with God's Spirit onto a wounded body.

9. Educate yourself outside of your specialty. Keep current with general medicine by scanning other literature. Visit the hospital library and browse journals you don't usually read. In addition, keep an eye on lay literature to see what current health issues are communicated to the public.

What is on the front page of the *Wall Street Journal, Time,* or *Ladies Home Journal*? What is the latest medical topic explored on the evening TV news – or on "Sixty Minutes"? Keep in mind that the media and reporters get journals just before release to public, so pay attention to medical issues in the public press. These may be the concerns brought to you the next day by your patient in the exam room.

It is also important to read non-medical literature to understand the human mind and heart. The world's great authors, including those of the Bible, can reveal human behavior that transcends time. Such reading will also help you know your patient in the context of the whole person. Always relate learning to real patients and real populations.

10. Always remember your God-given commission. You are a member of the body of Christ – you are there to serve, to heal, to comfort. You have the privilege of knowing the individual or the community in a unique and intimate way. Treasure this calling!

11. Develop tools for rapid reference in your office. Many Internet sites and software programs can help you find information quickly for urgent problems. A filing system for articles collected over the past five years, indexed in the computer, can be invaluable in keeping you up to date with problems you encounter in a busy clinic.

12. Practice the excellence you develop. Remember that all you learn must be converted into healing by your actions. Healing occurs when excellence and love are poured out with God's Spirit onto a wounded body. Practicing excellence means following through with all you have learned for the sake of the patient before you. It means avoiding shortcuts, doing a rectal exam even though you are certain the bleeding is from hemorrhoids.

Excellence means going back at the end of your day to check that disoriented patient, even though the nurses should call you if there are additional problems. Excellence means spending all the time the patient really needs in the examining room, even though thousands more wait outside. Excellence means reviewing the literature over a difficult problem rather than "shooting from the hip" of your memory. The practice of excellence involves willing yourself to do all that it takes to transform the knowledge you have gained into the health of your patient. Gain excellence—then practice it!

13. Take care of yourself. No one can practice excellence in medicine or dentistry if they are sleep-deprived, in poor shape physically, or burdened by worries at home. Be certain that you are doing what it takes to maximize your physical, emotional, and family well-being—or your patients will suffer from your distraction and fatigue.

Overwhelmed? This is when we need to do what we can while turning to God for his help. Determine to take one positive step and pray for God to multiply your efforts.

> "Whatever your task, work heartily, as serving the Lord and not men, knowing that from the Lord you will receive the inheritance as your reward; you are serving the Lord Christ" (Col. 3:23-24 RSV).

This is a scriptural call for excellence. Our excellence in our medical and public health endeavors can serve as a light to Christ for others and can be the platform on which we have influence for him in his name. We are given these opportunities to help build his kingdom in the hearts and lives of others.

THREE QUESTIONS TO ASK YOURSELF
1. Am I at the level of excellence in my work that God desires?
2. Where is there time in my life that could be used for improving my practice of medicine or dentistry through study? Should I drop an activity of lesser importance to allow that study?
3. How can God use my special area of excellence to speak his word of redemption?

THREE ACTIONS TO CONSIDER
1. Establish a mentor or mentoring group that you can meet with quarterly to review scientific advances and practice applications.
2. Schedule consistent time each week for personal study or educational conferences.
3. Find an avenue to use your knowledge as a teacher, writer, or as a speaker.

The practice of excellence involves willing yourself to do all that it takes to transform the knowledge you have gained into the health of your patient.

PRAYER

Oh, Lord, who embodies divine excellence, may we reflect you as our Creator by being excellent in each task that you set before us. Thank you for making us your workmanship and for the privilege of service in your name. May all that we do bring healing and health to those individual patients for whom we care, for those populations in our charge, for those inquiring minds that we may teach, and for those who would benefit from our efforts wherever that may be. May we model ourselves after you and in so doing, may we light the way for others to find you and know you in a deeper way, with joy.

–Amen

CHAPTER 5

Clinical Practice

"For no one can lay any foundation other than the one already laid, which is Jesus Christ" (1 Cor. 3:11).

When our oldest daughter was in her senior year of high school, we prayerfully sought out which colleges and universities we should visit as a family. Since she was interested in the nursing profession, we chose four Christian colleges that provided an opportunity for her to pursue a nursing degree. We picked our weekends to visit, arranged our schedules, and made a list of some standard questions to ask during our visits.

Being a Christian doctor, and interested in the integration of faith into the healthcare education curriculum, I decided to query professors in the nursing department of each college as to how the Christian faith influenced the nursing curriculum. I was determined to see that my daughter received an education with a Christian world view, unlike the secular education that I had received during undergraduate and medical school.

During one campus visit, I asked the chairperson of the nursing department, "How do you integrate principles of the Christian faith into the educational curriculum?" The woman who chaired the department, with a doctorate in nursing, looked at me as if somewhat surprised by my question. She responded, "I don't think you understand how we structure our curriculum here. There is only one foundation, and that is our Christian faith. Therefore, we integrate our healthcare curriculum into our Christian faith. Healthcare is a ministry founded on our Christian faith, not the other way around."

Although I don't remember that professor's name, I will never forget the lesson she taught me – all of life, no matter what our chosen vocation, should flow out of our relationship with God through Christ, as he is indeed the only foundation: "For in him we live and move and have our being..." (Acts 17:28).

—Steve Sartori M.D.

It is not what we do that determines who we are, but rather it is who we are that determines what we do.

Are we doctors who happen to be Christians or are we Christians whom God has called to be doctors? Does the answer to this question change when we walk through our office doors? Is one description like a sports coat we wear at home and the other like the white coat that identifies us as we face our patients and colleagues? The greatest challenge for us as Christian doctors today is our integration of the presence of Christ into our everyday practice as doctors. How we accomplish this integration will vary with our models of clinical and academic practice, but certain principles apply across the medical and dental disciplines that can guide us in this most essential endeavor. These principles begin with the clear understanding that it is not what we do that determines who we are, but rather it is who we are that determines what we do. Attitudes impact actions; beliefs determine behavior; character affects conduct; and, doctrine produces deeds. This is true for our lives at home and it is absolutely true for our lives at the office. So how do we go about converting this understanding into practical life guidelines?

MISSION STATEMENT

Do you have a personal mission statement for your practice as a doctor? Just as many of us have a personal mission statement or "life verse," our medical practices should also have a mission or purpose statement. One family practice group in eastern Kentucky has chosen the phrase "ministering the love of God through healthcare." This statement appears on their letterhead and business cards, and is a regular reminder of their reason for taking care of patients They want their patients to have the opportunity to experience the love of God as they come in contact with the medical practice. A personal mission statement reminds you who you are and why you go to work each day. Take the time, write one out, and then post it on your office wall.

CORE VALUES

As Christian doctors, we can formulate and articulate a set of values or principles defining the context within which we make decisions. For the Christian doctor, these values or principles should be based upon the Scriptures. The Christian group mentioned above has developed a set of seven core values or principles that guide their decision making and strategic planning:

◆MINISTRY: *"Jesus went through all the towns and villages, teaching in their synagogues, preaching the good news of the kingdom and healing every disease and sickness" (Matt. 9:35).*

For the Christian physician or healthcare professional, healthcare is a ministry, an opportunity to serve people and simultaneously expand the church of Jesus Christ. The ministry of Jesus included teaching, preaching, and healing. In Scripture the word for "save" and "heal" is essentially the same because the two are inextricably linked. Each patient we see has a 100 percent mortality rate, and there is only one physician who can cure their disease of sin–the Great Physician, Jesus Christ. His specialty is eternal medicine. The deepest need of patients who do not know Christ is to receive the gift of salvation by grace through faith in Jesus. For Christian patients, there is a need for instruction and encouragement in the application of biblical truth in every area of their lives.

♦**MEDICINE**: *"And wherever he went—into villages, towns or countryside—they placed the sick in the marketplaces. They begged him to let them touch even the edge of his cloak, and all who touched him were healed"* (Mark 6:56).

As physicians, we have been called to a vocation of caring for the sick. Patients have entrusted us with their healthcare, and it is a privilege to be granted this honor and responsibility. Just as Scripture encourages us to study and work to understand the Word of God (2 Tim. 2:15), similarly, we should study and work to achieve and maintain competence in our vocation. Excellence in our profession often yields the privilege of being heard by patients and colleagues not only on healthcare topics but also regarding spiritual issues, whereas a lack of competency will be likely to distract from our potential to be influential in the lives of patients and colleagues.

♦**MISSIONS**: *"Therefore go and make disciples of all nations, baptizing them in the name of the Father and of the Son and of the Holy Spirit, and teaching them to obey everything I have commanded you..."* (Matt. 28:19-20).

Jesus advised his followers shortly before his departure from this earth that they would be his witnesses, both locally and around the world (Acts 1:8). This prompts us to use healthcare as a means by which we can share the gospel and help make disciples, both locally and around the world.

Both short-term and long-term international medical service opportunities are available, as well as domestic opportunities. Short-term and long-term opportunities opportunities are available for doctors who hear the call to missions. The medical mission team provides an impetus for church growth, evangelistic opportunities with patients, and outreach to unbelieving healthcare professionals. Participants usually report personal spiritual growth, and often pursue additional short- or long-term medical missions

Patients have entrusted us with their healthcare, and it is a privilege to be granted this honor and responsibility.

Mentoring refers to not just teaching or transferring factual knowledge or procedural skills, but also to modeling character and leading by example.

work. CMDA offers access to a variety of missions-related work, including short-term opportunities through Global Health Outreach, opportunities in academic settings through Medical Education International, and long-term domestic opportunities guided by our Domestic Missions Commission.

♦**Mentoring**: *"You then, my son, be strong in the grace that is in Christ Jesus. And the things you have heard me say in the presence of many witnesses entrust to reliable men who will also be qualified to teach others"* (2 Tim. 2:1-2).

Mentoring refers to not just teaching or transferring factual knowledge or procedural skills, but also to modeling character and leading by example. Although most healthcare students receive adequate instruction in the scientific aspects of medicine, many are woefully lacking in the spiritual training necessary for effective ministry. As Christian physicians, we have the privilege and responsibility of teaching and training the next generation of healthcare providers. As we instruct them, we are investing not only in their lives, but also in the lives of their future students—in other words, mentoring is a ministry of multiplication, which will be covered more fully later in this book.

♦**Marriage and family**: *"He must manage his own family well and see that his children obey him with proper respect"* (1 Tim 3:4).

Unless our family life is well managed, the effectiveness of endeavors outside of the family may be compromised. In order to serve others effectively, it is imperative that our personal lives and relationships be in order. When the family relationships of the physician are good, then the physician is not distracted or preoccupied in ways that might detract from providing optimum patient care.

The marriage relationship is primary in any family. Marriage partners must make deliberate decisions to nurture this key relationship. Time must be committed to one another for prayer, communication, intimacy, ministry, and family activities. The best thing that parents can do for their children is to demonstrate their love for God and their love and unconditional commitment to one another. Living in an era and culture where the disintegration of the family is the norm and convenience rather than commitment drive relationships, it is important for Christian medical families to be distinctive and enduring.

♦**Margin**: *"There is a time for everything, and a season for every activity under heaven"* (Eccl. 3:1).

The healthcare landscape today is littered with the lives of burned out physicians. Thankfully, the Scriptures also give us the prescription for combating burnout and battle fatigue. Isaiah 40:31 says: "...but those who hope in the LORD will renew their strength. They will soar on wings like eagles; they will run and not grow weary, they will walk and not be faint." As we trust the Lord to be our refuge and strength, he will prove sufficient to meet our every need.

The Christian physician must deliberately choose to prioritize a daily time of prayer, Bible study, and devotions. Each activity opportunity should be scrutinized in order to evaluate its eternal importance. Strategic decisions should be made, choosing fewer activities with greater focus and intensity. Investments in the ministry of the local church should be focused in the areas of spiritual giftedness. Family vacations and mission trips should be planned and enjoyed. Deliberately allowing some unscheduled down time can represent opportunities for spontaneity and Spirit-led choices.

*MONEY: *"For where your treasure is, there your heart will be also" (Matt. 6:21).*

"For where your treasure is, there your heart will be also" (Matt. 6:21).

Principles related to money are last because decisions should be made on the basis of principles other than economics. We cannot serve both God and money (Matt. 6:24). We know that God created everything and has authority over all of his creation, and in reality possesses everything. We are merely entrusted with managing some of his assets. Our management reflects the values in our hearts.

Many times money achieves a higher degree of importance than it deserves. There is frequently tension between the ministry aspects of healthcare and the economic requirements necessary to continue the ministry. Ministry decisions may dictate our provision of care for the underinsured, uninsured, indigent and homeless with reduced or no reimbursement, whereas overhead costs require sufficient revenues to continue serving patients and providing incomes for employees and doctors.

Christian doctors should make stewardship and lifestyle decisions that minimize or eliminate debt and thereby maximize giving to the work of the church. They should minimize personal economic stress, thereby allowing maximum flexibility in work decisions, always being ready to hear and obey God as he leads us in the work to do, wherever and whenever he calls.

STRATEGIC PLANNING

With God's sovereignty in view, a strategic plan should be developed by each medical and dental practice, consistent with the mission, vision, and values of the particular practice. Whether that practice is distinctly

*The most
essential
component
of our
expression
of faith
in our
practices
is our
commitment
as doctors
to verbalize
that faith.*

Christian or not, the plan should involve a ministry plan, a healthcare plan, and a business plan with a budget. The integrated master plan should establish specific goals and objectives for each area, with specific tasks and deadlines. Accountability should involve regular evaluations and reviews, with revisions as indicated. Periodically, outside consultation from individuals or organizations should be considered. The strategic plan should address each component of your practice.

MINISTRY PLAN

The ministry plan should address issues such as creating and maintaining an appropriate office environment to reflect your ministry, establishing cooperative relationships with local churches and church leaders, and providing spiritual care for patients and staff members, utilizing prayer, the gospel, and biblical counseling. The ministry plan should also include discussions of specific moral and ethical healthcare issues, medical missions opportunities, and the provision of healthcare services for uninsured, underinsured, and indigent patients. *Ministry* is a word that may seem out of place in a secular practice, but Christian doctors should attempt to convince their secular colleagues of their responsibility toward the economically deprived and underinsured.

The medical office environment can demonstrate the faith and values of the practice in many ways, starting with the interactions between staff and patients. Staff members should be cordial and helpful to every patient. Patients should be treated with courtesy and respect at all times. Comforting and calming music can be utilized in the reception area and for the telephone system. Reading materials can be chosen to communicate Christian values and principles. Information regarding local church events can be posted in the reception area. Examination rooms might contain a Bible and a Christian news magazine.

The most essential component of our expression of faith in our practices is our commitment as doctors to verbalize that faith:

Several years ago, I became convinced that although our practice was known in the community as a Christian practice, with many noticeable signs of the faith of the physicians, I was not actively seeing the practice as a ministry.

I would occasionally pray with a patient, or encourage church attendance, but that was about the limit of my spiritual care. I could not identify many patients who had been referred to the Great Physician, Jesus Christ. I decided to attend a conference on healthcare evangelism.

At the conference, I was exposed to some new ideas about taking a spiritual history and praying with patients. I was also encouraged to share the gospel with patients who express interest and grant permission. During the conference, I made a personal commitment to be more intentional about routinely incorporating a spiritual history into my patient encounters. I also prayed for an opportunity to share the gospel with a patient, and that I would be more alert to opportunities for spiritual interventions during patient encounters.

Shortly after returning from the conference, I saw Edith during a follow-up visit. Edith was an elderly woman with multiple medical problems. She had been hospitalized several times over the prior year with congestive heart failure, and had even required assisted ventilation during several stays in the ICU. In our part of the country, we referred to her as being "bad sick."

After addressing her medical problems, I reminded Edith of how sick she had been recently, and how often she had been very close to death. I asked her if she had thought about death and what might happen to her should that occur, and she said she hadn't really paid much thought to it. After sharing briefly some of my personal testimony, I asked her if she would like to hear what the Bible said about eternal life. She eagerly granted me permission, and at the end of our visit, she expressed in her own words through prayer an understanding of God's plan of salvation.

Several days later, on a Saturday morning, I went to the local college gymnasium to play basketball with some of my partners. During the warm up time, Dave, my partner who was on call for the weekend, informed me that Edith had been in the Emergency Department the evening before and that this time she had not survived.

With tears in my eyes, I told him that only days before, during her last office visit, she had expressed a clear understanding and acceptance of God's salvation by grace through faith in Christ.

When I attended the visitation before her funeral, I asked her family members how she had been during the last days of her life. One of her daughters told me that although in the past she usually had been very grouchy, which I had to acknowledge as true, Edith had been exceptionally happy during the days since her last office visit. She had expressed to several of her family members, "My doctor has become a preacher."

This experience in my life firmly established my conviction that the gospel message is both important and urgent in the lives of our patients.

—Steve Sartori M.D.

As Christian doctors we should be committed to verbalizing our faith.

One of the best decisions we've ever made—for both staff and patients—was to involve a chaplain in our practice.

Equipping national healthcare providers with both medical and spiritual skills is a strategic investment in the kingdom of God.

In relation to your ministry plan, it is important to **develop good relationships with pastors and churches in your community**, as they often provide valuable resources for your patients. Lay health volunteers from the local church community can be utilized to make home visits focused on health education and evangelism. Other church volunteers may wish to come into the office setting to offer prayer support for patients in the practice. Local churches may wish to host healthcare screenings or clinics for the uninsured.

Another method of addressing the spiritual needs of patients and staff is to **involve a biblical counselor or chaplain** with the medical practice:

A few years ago, the doctors in our medical group practice decided to utilize a chaplain. A local pastor who was familiar with our medical group, whose life and family gave testimony to his deep and consistent faith walk with God, had a growing interest in biblical counseling and was pursuing additional training. When he was approached about becoming a chaplain for our practice, the time was opportune for us and him to see our ministry desires realized. He now provides spiritual encouragement and consultation for our doctors and staff, as well as intensive biblical counsel for some of our patients. I am convinced that this has been one of the best decisions we have ever made, as evidenced by the testimonies of many of our patients who have found freedom from depression, anxiety, relational rifts, and the bondage of besetting sin.

—Steve Sartori M.D.

Christian physicians can provide consultation to the local church, offering guidance on healthcare issues, especially relating to the difficult ethical issues of our day. Christian doctors can offer their services to speak to local churches on bioethical issues. Material to provide such instruction is readily available on the CMDA website. Churches may need assistance in understanding and establishing biblical healthcare models, such as calling the elders for prayer, and utilizing benevolent programs to assist with skyrocketing healthcare costs. In addition, several Christian healthcare cost sharing plans now provide alternative strategies to traditional health insurance plans.

Many of our patient encounters require practical decisions regarding moral and ethical issues. These decisions should be discussed and researched, and most importantly bathed in prayer and scriptural principles. Although Christian physicians may come to different conclusions and thereby implement different practice patterns regarding some of these ethical issues based on issues of conscience, practice partners can be invaluable in helping to come to conclusions regarding some of these difficult issues. Prov. 27:17 says: "As iron sharpens iron, so one man sharpens another."

The provision of **healthcare services to the poor and underserved** is part of our calling as Christian physicians. The Bible is replete with instructions to give generously to the poor, and providing healthcare services is one way to obey this instruction. God has chosen the poor to be rich in faith and to inherit his kingdom (James 2:5). Therefore, in serving the poor we are often serving our brothers and sisters in the true faith. Our loving service often yields opportunities for instruction, development, and empowerment in the lives of these patients, rather than merely relief and an entitlement syndrome.

A ministry plan may include **provision to pursue short-term medical missions opportunities**, either international or domestic. If you are in a group practice, coverage for patients can be arranged (for some it may require vacation time to do so). Some practices provide two weeks off annually for physicians to take a short-term medical mission trip. Short-term mission trips can be funded personally, or with the partnership of the local church or another supportive sponsoring organization. Although the personal cost in time and financial resources can be high, the rewards are great, and participants often repeat the experience.

I have participated with a healthcare mission in Romania for many years. Before one of our trips, we planned and organized an academic conference on gastrointestinal disease, including a practical preceptorship opportunity for endoscopy training. The short-term medical mission team included several primary care physicians, and two Christian gastroenterologists. Used endoscopy equipment and supplies were purchased with charitable contributions and personally transported by members of the mission team. After a tiresome and complicated process of customs clearance, the equipment was ultimately transported to the local hospital and set up in an operating suite. Miraculously, all of the equipment was operational, and all of the necessary supplies were available.

Two days of practical endoscopy training yielded excellent collegial relationships between the Romanian surgeons and the American gastroenterologists. Subsequently, an academic teaching conference was hosted for many of the physicians in the community. Along with the presentation of current information about gastrointestinal disease and other topics of interest, the missionary physicians were able to share about their personal faith in Jesus Christ. On the final evening of the conference, the Jesus video was shown in the Romanian language.

After this, one of the American physicians was able to share the gospel with the chief of surgery at the local hospital, who had been one of his students during the two days of endoscopy training. This popular and influential surgeon expressed his understanding of the gospel that evening, and professed faith in God's salvation

Patient needs should guide decisions to expand services or recruit additional providers.

It is difficult to overstate the impact that a rotation with a doctor who truly lives out the Christian faith can have on a student or resident.

plan. The following morning, he finished rounds early in order to attend a worship service at the Christian clinic.

The opportunities for this Romanian national physician to share the gospel with his own people will far exceed any opportunities provided an American doctor during a short-term medical mission trip. Equipping national healthcare providers with both medical and spiritual skills is a strategic investment in the kingdom of God.

–Steve Sartori M.D.

EMPLOYEES AND CO-WORKERS

"Whoever wants to become great among you must be your servant, and whoever wants to be first must be your slave–just as the Son of Man did not come to be served, but to serve, and to give his life as a ransom for many." (Matt. 10:26-28).

Though sad, it is rightly said that we tend to abuse those closest to us. While they might be our family and friends, for physicians and dentists, they are often our employees and others we oversee. We all know stories of doctors who are verbally abusive to nurses or hospital staff. While some of these doctors may be Christians, they are not acting like Christ. There are times when each of us may fall short in the way we treat those who work with us.

Passages from Philemon and Paul's pastoral letters make it clear that we have great responsibility for those under our authority – not only to be a fair employer, but also to be an effective witness and example of Christ. One Christian doctor surveyed her staff to learn what characteristics they have seen in Christian doctors. While some of the responses were flattering, not all were, including these: "no joy," "too rushed," "failing to show appreciation," "jumping to conclusions," and "lying." Ouch!

Remember, the opportunity to influence (positively and negatively) those under our authority may be greater for staff and fellow workers than for patients. We must not shirk our responsibility to do so. "In the same way, let your light shine before men, that they may see your good deeds and praise your Father in heaven" (Matt. 5:16).

HEALTHCARE PLAN

How do Christian doctors determine such issues as group size, location of services, and the types of services that they will provide for their community? Patient needs should guide decisions to expand services or recruit additional providers. If there are medical services needed in your community that fall within the realm of your skill and training, then these services should probably be offered. If other providers in the community are offering quality service and fulfilling your community's need for a particular service, it may be wise not to duplicate services and to focus on other areas of need. If patient needs or desires for a certain quality of healthcare are not being met in the community, then the recruitment of additional professional providers should be pursued.

Although many Christian physicians are salt and light in secular medical practices, they should be prayerfully concerned about being united in partnership or ownership with nonbelievers. Since Christians are advised to not be yoked together with unbelievers (2 Cor. 6:14), Christian physicians should consider recruiting like-minded fellow believers to serve together with them. This is not always possible, nor is it always God's will. CMDA has an excellent recruitment service.

Inviting premedical students, medical students, and residents into your practice is a means of demonstrating the ministry model of healthcare first hand. These students will increase their medical knowledge and skills, learn spiritual care skills, and also observe your professional and personal relationships. Although this can be intimidating, this apprenticeship model of teaching is highly effective. Some doctors have attempted to include students in their family activities by providing housing or extending meal invitations, or by including them in activities such as sporting events, sightseeing, or church attendance. At the end of the rotation a gift such as a Bible or a copy of the book *The Faith Factor* might be provided as a reminder of their experience during their rotation. It is difficult to overstate the impact that a rotation with a doctor who truly lives out the Christian faith can have on a student or resident.

What are your hours going to be? Will you have any nights or weekend clinics? Are you going to allow walk-ins or add-ons?

A personal friend of mine asked if his daughter, who was interested in a healthcare career, could spend a couple of weeks with our practice. We hosted her in our home, and I included her in the usual activities of a small-town family practice doctor in group practice. She accompanied me during each of my patient encounters, and I sought to provide teaching points related to the particular visit. During the first week of her rotation, after dinner in our home, I overheard her in our guest bedroom talking with her father on the telephone.

"Dad, you won't believe what happened in the office today!" she said. "A patient prayed to receive Christ as their Savior!" Obviously, this experience was the primary impression from her day at the office, and left an indelible imprint in her life experience about the role of healthcare evangelism.

–Steve Sartori M.D.

BUSINESS PLAN

American medicine has become complicated by **administrative requirements imposed upon practices**, which make it difficult to maximize patient

Physicians are in the unusual business situation of facing increasing costs and unfunded regulatory burdens without the usual option of increasing revenues through increased fees.

care, minimize error, and maximize financial productivity. At least the following areas are affected:

♦**Scheduling**. In the area of scheduling, it is most important to be honest, realistic, and practical. The key person to making a schedule work is the physician. Thus it is important to do an honest self-assessment. Ask yourself: *Am I a person who is on time?* If yes, great. If not, then why not and can you change? Next ask yourself about your own proclivities and preferences. For example – when do you want off; when do you want to see new patients, when do you want to see follow-up patients – and other related questions. Other relevant questions revolve around accessibility for your patients: What are your hours going to be? Will you have any nights or weekend clinics? Are you going to allow walk-ins or add-ons? You also need to ask yourself how many patients you need to see to achieve your desired income. All of this information should then be sifted to develop the scheduling templates for the practice.

♦**Patient Information**. It is absolutely vital that the patient information and insurance information be accurately obtained and maintained. It is strongly suggested that at least every six months, or at every encounter, a practice present patients with a printout of their demographic and insurance information, asking them to update it if necessary. These changes should be entered into the computer system immediately.

♦**Benefits**. In some specialties it is very important to verify the actual insurance benefits that patients have before their first encounter with the physician. This may prevent some very difficult situations, for example, the occasion of a patient's insurer denying payment on a major service so that the patient is left with the responsibility a large bill.

♦**Precertification**. The whole precertification/preauthorization process should be followed to ensure that patients are approved for any treatments or procedures. The staff should be trained in this area. The best practices create a one page sheet for each payer's requirements for precert, diagnostic, and lab work to ensure that a patient's care will be paid for by the insurer.

♦**Co-pays**. Know the patient's co-pay and collect it at the time of service. When the insurance carrier set up the plan and set the physician's reimbursement rate for care, it established a cost-sharing mechanism via co-pays and assumed that the doctor's office would collect these to ensure that the revenue from the plan was sufficient for the physician to be in the payer's panel. The doctors in a practice have a moral obligation to follow the terms of co-pay that were committed to in signing up with a given insurer.

◆**Transcription & Medical Records**. There is no right way to do this – just the way that works best for you. The most important part is that it needs to be done and it needs to be accurate and current. The physician should try to complete his/her dictation each clinic day. It is critical to have a staff person or dictation service that can turn this work around within twenty-four to forty-eight hours. Then have your staff ensure that the charts are kept current.

FINANCIAL OPERATIONS

The practice of medicine entails a significant financial stewardship. For nearly all physician practices this stewardship differs little from a typical household budget – it runs month to month, or even week to week. There are so many important details that all must be done well in order to maintain a sound financial state within a medical practice. This section will address several of those areas:

◆**Budget**. It is amazing how many medical practices do not work on a budget. A budget is a basis for any financial plan. The Medical Group Management Association (MGMA) and the American Medical Association (AMA) have template resources as well as more detailed material to assist your practice in developing a realistic budget.

◆**Accounts Receivable**. A consistent flow of accounts receivable is essential to any medical practice. The key to this success is two-fold: good people and good processes. It is imperative that this aspect of your practice maintain as much commitment to excellence as any aspect on the clinical side. The fundamental principle for successful accounts receivable is to keep everything current. Today's charges should be posted no later than tomorrow. Today's checks should be posted today. Claims should be electronically submitted (or submitted on paper) daily. Accounts should be worked to minimize balances over sixty days. Low payments, non-payments, bundling, and other insurance company schemes should be challenged persistently. Everyone involved in the billing department should be cross-trained to ensure that there are no disruptions in the work flow.

Those of us who are followers of Christ must pray about the difficult area of patient debt and seek first to honor God both in our discussions and in our decision making.

One of the most challenging tasks a doctor faces is that of hiring and retaining excellent employees.

Decisions must be made in every practice regarding charges for services and collection of patient debt. In the healthcare environment today, there is progressive economic pressure as expenses continue to increase while the market and revenues are limited by third party payers.

Physicians are in the unusual business situation of facing increasing costs and unfunded regulatory burdens without the usual option of increasing revenues through increased fees. These pressures make it even more important to manage resources carefully.

Practice revenues are highly variable depending upon patient volume, procedures performed, and contractual adjustments and the competency and perseverance of staff members dedicated to the billing and collections functions within the medical practice. Policies regarding patients who do not pay their medical bills should reflect the values of the organization.

When patients do not pay their bills, many Christian doctors do not transfer the responsibility of dealing with this issue to a collection agency, since a collection agency may not represent their corporate values. Instead, such practices attempt to personally contact patients who have not paid their account in a timely fashion, so as to determine the individual circumstances.

In many cases, debts are forgiven or reduced. Some patients agree to a budget plan. In some cases, patients are forgiven of debt, but denied the privilege of future medical care. These patients are informed of this by certified letter. (See a sample policy and letter at the end of this chapter.)

In discussions with our associates, each of us must decide our approach to patient debt. Those of us who are followers of Christ must pray about this difficult area and seek first to honor God both in our discussions and in our decision making.

♦**Accounts Payable**. Paying bills in a timely manner is a commitment to which all Christians should adhere. By using a budget, a medical practice can be faithful to its moral obligation, good credit, and public testimony by paying its bills and debts on time.

♦**Payroll**. One of the largest expenses in any medical practice is the employee payroll, taxes, and benefits. Christians should pay their staff a fair wage. In order to determine whether this is the case, a physician may have to obtain a salary survey for their community. Often local medical societies have this information. If this is not available, then the local chapter of the Medical Group Management Association may be able to assist.

+**Capital (Future) Investment**. The principle of setting aside for future growth provides more flexibility than having to borrow for growth and development. Christians have different views on the latter, some believing that they should never borrow and others believing that borrowing is acceptable, within limits. One reality is true: "...the borrower is servant to the lender" (Prov. 22:7). Thus, managed savings for adding another physician or more staff or more services or new equipment or another facility is the more prudent approach to building toward the future.

HUMAN RESOURCES

Human Resources envelops hiring, training, retention, policies and procedures, discipline, evaluation, development and promotion.

+**Hiring**. One of the most challenging tasks a doctor faces is that of hiring and retaining excellent employees. In addition to seeking specific technical skills required for a position, we all seek employees who possess **enthusiasm**, **eagerness to learn**, **unselfishness**, and the **high moral standards** normally associated with personal faith. The best employees do not need constant supervision but are motivated to strive for excellence by their own character or by their dedication to the Lord. Ideally, those you hire will live by the principle expressed in Col. 3:23, "Whatever you do, do your work heartily, as for the Lord rather than for men" (NASB).

Humility is also crucial in a good employee. Employees who are humble will be a joy to their fellow employees, and will also be open to learning new and better ways of doing things. They will receive constructive criticism with open arms; their competence will continue to grow throughout their professional careers; and they will more consistently treat your patients with respect and compassion.

Of course, you cannot hope to hire only dedicated followers of Christ in most practice situations; but it is crucial that employees endorse moral stardards consistent with your practice's core values and mission. The closer your employees' own values complement your practice's values and mission, the more likely it is that they will be achieved.

How can you learn about a potential employee's spiritual status without breaking any civil laws? Any prospective employee has the right to know in advance the philosophical basis by which the practice operates. A conscientious employer will, at some point during the interview process, inform the potential employee of this foundational practice information. It might go something like this: "Miss Jones, in order for you to determine whether or not this is the right position for you, I want you to know as

Do not hire just anyone for a position, and certainly don't hire someone because they are a family member, friend, or acquaintance.

Although there are no passages that specifically deal with how to fire an employee, the Scriptures do contain foundational principles of accountability which are instructive in this regard.

much as you can about our practice. I am a Christian and the Bible is the guide for everything I do in life. For this reason, all policies in our office - our appointment book policy, our financial policy, our employee policies, our standard operating procedures - are based upon my understanding of the teachings of the Bible. Would you be comfortable working in such an environment?" The response will help you decide whether the person is spiritually compatible with your office work plan.

In addition to these qualities, as we interview prospective employees, we should consider **seven additional factors**, each starting with the letter C. These words are character, competency, cooperation, communication, compassion, commitment, and consistency. **Character** flows from the beliefs and values of the individual, and is something that cannot be taught. **Competency** causes us to examine individual giftedness, skills, and experience. **Cooperation** stresses the importance of being able to establish and maintain encouraging and collaborative working relationships as members of the same team. **Communication** refers to the ability to communicate effectively both by spoken and written word. **Compassion** is a core virtue as a worker in a medical practice. **Commitment** refers to the loyalty of the individual to the organization. **Consistency** means that the person exhibits behavior that is in line with stated values and beliefs.

When recruiting staff, the most important issue to discern is whether or not the individual shares the organizational mission, vision, and values. A person who shares these core values is a "mission match." Open-ended questions can be formulated that invite potential employees to express their values, as well as the origin of those value systems. Do not hire just anyone for a position, and certainly don't hire someone because they are a family member, friend, or acquaintance. This is one of the most common problems in physician practices. There are some basic practical matters that can really ensure that you hire the right person for the job. These include: writing a job description, conducting a thorough interview, interviewing multiple candidates, and contacting references.

♦**Training**. Physician practices are renowned for implementing a "sink or swim" attitude with their staff. Depending on the size of the practice and the complexity of the job, it is strongly suggested that each employee be put through a one- to three-week training program. Key items that should be addressed in a training program include: general information about the practice, policies and procedures, job description and details, cross training, and employee benefits.

• **Retention.** It is very costly to lose an employee. Thus it is important to learn the key elements necessary to keep employees. An annual assessment of key elements of retention is important for the practice. These elements may include: a salary survey, benefit survey, work conditions survey, morale survey, and a competition survey.

• **Policies and Procedures.** Employees should know the standards by which their performance will be evaluated. Such standards should be available in a job description, an office policy manual, treatment protocol, and other documentation, so employees will know what is expected of them. Written policies and procedures are vital to ensuring fairness, compliance, and morale among the staff. An employee handbook addressing issues such as vacation, sick leave, bereavement, benefits, payroll policies, attendance, discipline, and so forth is key to ensuring that all staff understand the rules of engagement that apply equally to all employees in the practice.

There should be periodic opportunities for employee reviews, so employees know where they stand, both with respect to praiseworthy accomplishments and areas of potential improvement. For new employees the frequency might be monthly or quarterly, but it would seem that all employees should have some type of formal review at least yearly. A system of periodic reviews does not preclude an employer from dealing with correctable events as they occur, but at least it guarantees that issues will be dealt with on some sort of regular basis.

• **Discipline.** Any doctor who plays a managerial role in his or her practice will at times come to the realization that a particular employee does not belong in the practice. This can be a traumatic event, for both the doctor and the employee. What do the Scriptures teach in this regard?

Although there are no passages that specifically deal with how to fire an employee, the Scriptures do contain foundational principles of accountability which are instructive in this regard. In Matt. 18:15-17, Jesus prescribes the pattern for approaching someone who is believed to be doing something wrong. He doesn't call for the most severe penalty (in this passage, excommunication) to be rendered as the first option. Rather, he calls for a one-on-one confrontation. If this is not successful, other steps are to follow, which could eventually result in excommunication. In a somewhat similar fashion, the employee whose performance is unacceptable should be informed of the area of concern, and should be given an opportunity to correct the deficiency.

Perhaps you've heard the secular advice that employees need to hear both praise and constructive criticism in order to improve. This works because it is a reflection of the wisdom of God.

In relation to this, it is vital to have a written, consistent, and enforced policy of employee discipline. This policy should address at least two categories of violations – minor infractions (tardiness) and major infractions (abuse, harassment, etc.). Minor infractions usually have an incremental disciplinary process. For example, in relation to tardiness: first infraction – verbal warning; second infraction – written warning; third infraction – final written warning; fourth infraction – termination.

Minor infractions should retain the opportunity to start fresh. For example, if an employee is tardy twice this year and has received a verbal and written warning, the clock is reset next year and the next tardy is considered the first tardy.

Major infractions usually result in final written warning or termination. For example, an employee who abuses a patient or fails to show up at work without calling in should receive very strict discipline.

The goal of all discipline should be to correct or improve performance – or in the uncorrectable situation to terminate an employee whose behavior is harming your practice.

♦**Evaluation.** Perhaps you've heard the secular advice that employees need to hear both praise and constructive criticism in order to improve. This works because it is a reflection of the wisdom of God. All employees will be praiseworthy to at least some extent, because they are image-bearers of God (Gen. 1:26). For this reason, an employer will always be able to find at least some elements of praise to bestow on each employee. Employers who do not take the time and interest to genuinely praise and encourage employees will likely find criticism falling on deaf ears.

Just as every employee reflects various aspects of the image of God, each will also possess and demonstrate imperfections related to the rebellion found in every human heart (Jer. 17:9). Hebrews 12:6 tells us "...the Lord disciplines those whom he loves..." (NASV). If we truly care about the ongoing development of our employees, we will offer correction when indicated, and we will do it in love. For an employer to critique an employee based upon standards that have not been communicated will be exasperating to the employee (Col. 3:21).

♦**Development and Promotion.** Many employees are interested in their own professional growth and development. A medical or dental practice should encourage its staff to excel through participation in programs, meetings, and organizations that equip the employee to be more skilled in their area of expertise. Ultimately, this commitment to excellence enhances the opportunity for promotion within the practice.

Our clinical practice: this is where we will most likely impact our world for Jesus Christ. Do we do it well? If we do, then God will have fulfilled much of his purpose for our lives. If we do it poorly, then let's decide to change.

THREE QUESTIONS TO ASK YOURSELF

1. Do I view my medical practice as a ministry?
2. How do my attitudes and actions demonstrate to others that I am a follower of Jesus?
3. What practical changes might God want me to make in my practice?

THREE ACTIONS TO CONSIDER

1. Write down a personal and practice mission statement, based upon at least one verse from Scripture.
2. Meet with at least one other Christian healthcare professional in order to pray for God's direction in your practice.
3. Develop a ministry plan that includes spiritual care for your patients.

PRAYER

Dear God and Father,
Thank you for Jesus, my Savior. Thank you for the Holy Spirit who lives in me. Thank you for the privilege of being a healthcare professional. I ask for your wisdom as I seek to bring honor and glory to you through the ministry of healthcare. Please reveal to me any changes you want me to make in my personal life and practice, and grant me the power to make these changes. May your kingdom come and your will be done, I pray, in the name of Jesus.

–Amen

SAMPLE COLLECTION POLICY AND LETTER

After making many errors in the way we tried to collect payments from patients, we finally developed a policy and procedure that seems to be God-honoring. The critical foundation for this policy and procedure was the collection philosophy: first understand what is going on in the life of the patient and why they have not fulfilled their responsibility, and then respond as Christ would.

The following letter would be sent only after a series of "routine" collection attempts. The third invoice would request that the patient contact the office if there was an error in the bill, if they were not pleased with the care they received, or if they have a personal need that has interfered with their ability to pay.

If there was no response and we could not reach the patient by phone, the following letter was sent by registered mail with a return receipt requested.

Dear <   >:

It is with sadness that I write this letter. I am only made aware of a patient's account status when it becomes an issue that affects our relationship. Such is now the case. My office manager has notified me of your failure to pay the debt incurred from the care we provided <you, your family, or individual>.

We take our responsibility to you seriously, and are concerned that we have not heard from you. I understand that the office staff has tried to contact you, hoping to solve any problems. We wanted to be sure the bill was correct and that you were pleased with our care. We also wanted to know if you were facing a problem that kept you from paying. In addition to our desire to give you excellent care, we are interested in you as a person – your concerns and needs. Only when we know about your situation can we adjust our expectations.

There may be other reasons we have not heard from you, but we must assume that you do not intend to fulfill your responsibility in our relationship. Therefore, after <date four weeks in advance> we will remove your name from our active patient list and no longer provide <you or family member> care. During this time I would advise that you seek to register with another <physician/dentist>. With written permission from you, we will forward copies of your records to the doctor you select.

As for the debt you owe, we would like to follow the example set by God. We all owe a debt to him. None of us can pay that debt. But God cared enough for us that he forgave our debt through Jesus Christ. While this forgiveness is offered to everyone, our relationship with him is only restored when we accept it on his terms. Following that example, we have forgiven your debt to us. However, our relationship has been broken and can only be restored if you are willing to discuss ways to re-establish the relationship on mutual trust and responsibility.

If you are interested in re-establishing your relationship with our practice, please call <person> at <phone number> to schedule a meeting time.

With concern,

<Doctor's name and signature>

CHAPTER 6

Our Responsibility for the Poor

Dave and Marilyn Ziegler decided to celebrate their thirty-sixth wedding anniversary with a trip to Branson, Missouri. They did not often take vacations and the last couple of years had been tough financially. Dave had transitioned from working in the insurance industry to a home-based telecommunications business. The start-up phase had been slower going than they had hoped.

In Branson on their first day, Dave seemed to struggle to keep up with Marilyn. On the second day, they decided to have lunch at a buffet restaurant near their hotel. Late in the meal, Dave abruptly got up from the table, presumably to get a cup of coffee. He returned, and, a few minutes later, collapsed on the floor in what looked like a seizure.

Paramedics arrived quickly and Marilyn watched them work vigorously to help revive Dave. Despite their concentrated efforts, he did not respond; Dave had suffered a fatal heart attack and died. Later, when she was given the contents of his pockets, Marilyn found a small bottle of nitroglycerin tablets. Dave had never told her that he had heart disease.

Marilyn returned home to face the difficult tasks associated with burying her husband. The funeral was well attended; Dave had been a faithful supporter of the youth ministry of their church and was well loved by many. When all those events were over, she quickly learned that her financial status was far worse than she'd anticipated. With the demands of raising their family, she and her husband had been unable to save much money over the years. By mutual agreement, Marilyn had not worked much outside their home; she had shouldered the primary responsibility of caring for their four children.

At the time of Dave's death, two of those children were still in college. Dave's life insurance policy was not adequate to secure Marilyn's previous way of life, and her children were struggling with young careers and families. Her long-time

The most influential doctor in history was not Hippocrates, Jenner, or Osler. The world's most influential doctor was a first century physician-turned-missionary named Luke.

friends at church were emotionally supportive during the initial shock, but neither they nor anyone in the church leadership inquired about her financial situation.

Before long, Marilyn's savings were gone. She had continued to pay high monthly rates to maintain her health insurance, but could only to do so for about eighteen months. When that coverage disappeared she was unable to afford any other private health insurance. With reluctance, she applied for and received Medicaid.

When she contacted the office of her long-time doctor, she was told that he did not participate in the Medicaid program because it paid so poorly. Despite the fact that she had seen this doctor for a number of years, she was advised to seek care elsewhere. Some time later she contacted the office of her dentist. She and her family had long received care from this Christian dentist who was a leader in Dave and Marilyn's church. The dentist's office manager informed Marilyn that if she no longer had insurance, she would be expected to pay full price for her dental care. When Marilyn asked for special consideration because of the established relationship and her recent loss, she was politely refused.

The most influential doctor in the history of the world was not Hippocrates, Jenner, or Osler. Beyond comparison, the world's most influential doctor was a first century physician-turned-missionary named Luke. The Apostle Paul wrote thirteen books of the Bible, John another five, but Luke's writings (his gospel and the book of Acts) make up more of the volume of the New Testament than either of them. Countless millions around the world have studied Luke's accounts of Jesus' ministry and the early church's history for twenty centuries. Combine the readerships of Drs. Spock, Atkins, even Dr. Seuss, and they don't come close. Luke is our most accomplished and widely published colleague. If we are interested in the Christian doctor's responsibility to the poor, we will do well to consult Dr. Luke.

Luke's gospel has some of the richest Greek in the Bible. It also features stories and passages not recorded anywhere else in the Scriptures. He alone gives us the full account of the events surrounding Jesus' birth, the story of Zacchaeus in the sycamore tree, the nine ungrateful lepers, and several unforgettable parables including the Good Samaritan and the Prodigal Son. In chapter one, he records two of the Bible's most beautiful poetic passages—Mary's Magnificat and Zechariah's Song.

The most pervasive theme in the Gospel of Luke is God's concern for the poor. That may seem like an overstatement, but the theme appears in fully half of the gospel's twenty-four chapters. (See abbreviated list below.) Matthew, Mark, and John record warnings about the dangers of greed and mandate our responsibility to share with the poor, but Luke devotes more material to these subjects than the other gospel writers.

Over and over, Luke proclaims God's favor toward the poor and a corresponding disfavor toward the selfishly rich.

- Chapter 1: Following the announcement from the angel Gabriel that she would bear the Christ, Mary declares, "He (the LORD) has filled the hungry with good things but has sent the rich away empty" (1:53).

- Chapter 2: Mary and Joseph bring the eight-day-old Jesus to the Temple for presentation before the Lord. Leviticus 12 commanded Jewish parents to offer a year-old lamb as a sacrifice for their firstborn son, but because they were poor, Mary and Joseph take advantage of a provision that permitted the substitution of two inexpensive birds. When God became part of the human race, he chose to do so within a poor family.

- Chapter 4: Jesus is rejected after teaching in his hometown synagogue in Nazareth. His teaching text was from Isa. 61: "The Spirit of the Lord is on me, because he has anointed me to preach good news to the poor. He has sent me to proclaim freedom for the prisoners and recovery of sight for the blind, to release the oppressed, to proclaim the year of the Lord's favor" (4:18-19). From the outset of his preaching, Jesus identified meeting the needs of the poor as central to his ministry.

- Chapter 6: This chapter contains Luke's complement to Matthew's Beatitudes. Luke has "blessed are you" sections like Matthew, but follows them up with corresponding curses. "But woe to you who are rich, for you have already received your comfort. Woe to you who are well fed now, for you will go hungry" (6:24-25).

- Chapter 8: In the parable of the sower, some of the sower's seeds fell among thorns, which choked the plants and kept them from bearing fruit. Jesus explains that some will not bear spiritual fruit because of their attachment to "...life's worries, riches and pleasures..." (8:14).

- Chapter 10: When asked by an expert in the Law, "And who is my neighbor?" (10:29), Jesus responds with a story about two Jewish religious figures, a priest and a Levite, who ignored the physical needs of a desperate fallen man. What the two seemingly righteous men failed to do was performed instead by a religiously suspect Samaritan who understood what "love your neighbor as yourself" meant.

Over and over, Luke proclaims God's favor toward the poor and a corresponding disfavor toward the selfishly rich.

The entire sixteenth chapter of Luke's gospel is about wealth, greed, and biblical justice.

- Chapter 12: When asked by someone in the crowd to get involved in a family money dispute (12:13), Jesus tells the story of a rich fool who hoarded his wealth at the cost of his soul.

- Chapter 14: In Luke's account of the parable of the great banquet, the master sends out his messengers to call those invited to the feast. One after another, they make excuses related to their possessions or their families. The master responds by rejecting the original invitees and, instead, bringing in "the poor, the crippled, the blind and the lame" (14:21).

- Chapter 18: In the familiar story of the rich young ruler who elects not to follow Jesus because of great wealth, Jesus responds, "How hard it is for the rich to enter the kingdom of God! Indeed, it is easier for a camel to go through the eye of a needle than for a rich man to enter the kingdom of God" (18:24-25).

- Chapter 19: Zacchaeus, the corrupt tax collector proves his conversion by promising to repay those from whom he has extorted money. Additionally, he proclaims, "Look, Lord! Here and now I give half of my possessions to the poor..." (19:8). Jesus responds to this pledge by saying, "Today salvation has come to this house...."

- Chapter 21: The poor widow's offering of less than a dollar is praised in contrast to the larger gifts of the rich who don't give sacrificially (21:1-4).

This list of texts would be impressive enough, but even more notable is the fact that the entire sixteenth chapter of Luke's gospel is about wealth, greed, and biblical justice. It begins with perhaps the most difficult to understand of all Jesus' parables–the parable of the shrewd manager (Luke 16:1-15). In this story, a corrupt household manager is commended because he leveraged the possessions of his employer for his own benefit. The teaching points are delivered in a two-punch combination. Punch one: "I tell you, use worldly wealth to gain friends for yourselves, so that when it is gone, you will be welcomed into eternal dwellings" (16:9). Punch two: "So if you have not been trustworthy in handling worldly wealth, who will trust you with true riches?" (16:11). Jesus urges his disciples to use all that he has given them on earth to maximize their treasure in heaven. Conversely, if disciples do not pursue that course, they disqualify themselves from receiving heavenly rewards.

Jesus concludes this story with the familiar statement, "You cannot serve both God and Money" (16:13). A group of Pharisees in the audience, because they loved money, sneered. Jesus, confronted with outwardly religious people who professed faithfulness to God but inwardly sought their own profit, had stinging words of rebuke: "You are the ones who justify yourselves in the eyes of men, but God knows your hearts. What is highly valued among men is detestable in God's sight" (16:15). Luke 16 ends with one of the most frightening stories in the Bible. The passage referred to as "the rich man and Lazarus" (16:19-31) is not a parable, symbolically comparing everyday things to spiritual reality; it is the tale of a particular man burning in hell:

> There was a rich man who was dressed in purple and fine linen and lived in luxury every day. At his gate was laid a beggar named Lazarus, covered with sores and longing to eat what fell from the rich man's table. Even dogs came and licked his sores.
>
> The time came when the beggar died and the angels carried him to Abraham's side. The rich man also died and was buried. In hell, where he was in torment, he looked up and saw Abraham far away, with Lazarus by his side. So he called to him, "Father Abraham, have pity on me and send Lazarus to dip the tip of his finger in water and cool my tongue, because I am in agony in this fire."
>
> But Abraham replied, "Son, remember that in your lifetime you received your good things, while Lazarus received bad things, but now he is comforted here and you are in agony. And besides all this, between us and you a great chasm has been fixed, so that those who want to go from here to you cannot, nor can anyone cross over from there to us."
>
> He answered, "Then I beg you, father, send Lazarus to my father's house, for I have five brothers. Let him warn them, so that they will not also come to this place of torment."
>
> Abraham replied, "They have Moses and the Prophets, let them listen to them."
>
> "No, father Abraham," he said, "but if someone from the dead goes to them, they will repent."
>
> He said to him, "If they do not listen to Moses and the Prophets; they will not be convinced even if someone rises from the dead" (Luke 16:19-31).

At first reading, this passage might seem problematic for Christians. Like the well-known story of the sheep and the goats in Matthew 25, Jesus seems to be teaching that individuals go to heaven or hell based on whether or not they met the needs of the poor. Recall the judgment pronounced upon the goats in Matthew 25:41-43:

If our salvation is by faith alone, why does it appear that some people are rejected because of their deeds, and specifically because they ignore the poor?

Luke was a brilliant man. It would be illogical to conclude that he unknowingly contradicted himself about something as important as the means of salvation.

Then he will say to those on his left, "Depart from me, you who are cursed, into the eternal fire prepared for the devil and his angels. For I was hungry and you gave me nothing to eat, I was thirsty and you gave me nothing to drink, I was a stranger and you did not invite me in, I needed clothes and you did not clothe me, I was sick and in prison and you did not look after me."

So why does Jesus tell stories like these? If our salvation is by faith alone, why does it appear that some people are rejected because of their deeds, and specifically because they ignore the poor? And what about the author, Luke? In the book of Acts he records sermons and teachings of the apostles that clearly teach salvation by faith alone. Luke was a brilliant man. It would be illogical to conclude that he unknowingly contradicted himself about something as important as the means of salvation.

We must conclude that if there appears to be an inconsistency in the teachings of Scripture, the fault lies with our capacity to understand and believe. Somehow the fact that God unilaterally saves people by his mercy through faith in Jesus Christ is not incompatible with others being rejected because of what they did or didn't do. But how can the two be reconciled? How do we reconcile the great biblical truth of salvation by faith and the teachings of Luke 16 and Matthew 25?

The most reasonable answer is that there actually is a tension but no contradiction. Salvation is by faith, without any additional merit added by good deeds. It begins and ends with God. Our best efforts at righteousness are entirely inadequate. Those who are recipients of God's gracious salvation, however, will certainly demonstrate a radical and growing obedience to the teachings of Jesus and the apostles. This visible obedience is not to earn favor with God or to secure our salvation in an ongoing way. In fact, our obedience and good works, including serving the poor, are only possible because God gives his Holy Spirit to those who have saving faith. It is the Spirit of God inside the believer that makes growing obedience and God-glorifying good deeds possible. Conversely, if there is an absence of a visible and growing obedience to the teachings of Jesus and the apostles in a professed believer's life, particularly toward serving the poor, then that person needs to examine the veracity of his or her salvation experience. For as Jesus said, "Why do you call me 'Lord, Lord,' and do not do what I say?" (Luke 6:46).

Neither Luke nor Paul are troubled by side-by-side statements indicating salvation is by faith and followed by, even "proven" by, good deeds. Both John Calvin and Martin Luther went to great lengths to point out that truly converted Christians must bear the fruit of good works, including generously serving the poor.

Martin Luther said: "We also confess, and have always better and more forcibly taught, that good works must be done; that they must follow faith, and that faith is dead if good works be absent."

So we can conclude that the Apostle Paul, the gospel writer Luke, and especially Jesus, teach us that true disciples will demonstrate the reality of their conversion by obeying the commandments of Jesus. We can further conclude from the Scriptures that generously meeting the needs of the poor is a vital and non-negotiable aspect of the true disciple's obedience.

By contrast, the story of the rich man and Lazarus portrays a man in hell because he lived in luxury while ignoring the needy. Yet, it is also a story about a man who went to hell because he did not have faith. He was guilty of both ignoring God's commands and not trusting in God's promises. He practiced neither obedience nor faith, and consequently his end was tragic and eternal.

PRACTICE BY THE BOOK

What does this mean for a Christian physician or dentist trying to be a disciple of Jesus? In this era of God's kingdom, we too must seek to obey and glorify our Lord by serving the poor. We must recognize that Jesus calls us to meet the needs of the unfortunate in ways that are consistent with and even greater than the commandments in the Law and the Prophets. This is not to be done purely out of duty, although we certainly have a duty to meet. It is not done to earn favor with God, although he is most worthy of our unquestioning obedience.

Rather, it is to be done in faith, in the power of the Holy Spirit, and ultimately out of love for our King and God-given love for our neighbors. It is to be done in faith that God will bless us as we obey; that God will provide what we need, materially and spiritually, as we take loving risks in generosity. This sort of faith will show the world around us that we value God and his promises more than the material possessions of Western culture. This sort of faith will teach our children the costs and the blessings of kingdom obedience. This sort of faith will mercifully meet the needs of the suffering and the poor, for the sake of Jesus. This sort of faith will ultimately gain us treasure in heaven, forever.

Our obedience begins with the recognition of some difficult facts. Back to Luke 16: "There was a rich man who was dressed in purple and fine linen and lived in luxury every day." The world has never seen a more prosperous country than the United States of America. Although we make up only 2.5 percent of the world's population, we have 40 percent of the world's

"We also confess, and have always better and more forcibly taught, that good works must be done; that they must follow faith, and that faith is dead if good works be absent."
—Martin Luther

Giving as a percentage among Americans, and specifically among Christians, has steadily dropped over the last fifty years, despite the fact that our relative earnings have markedly grown.

wealth. While physicians and dentists have seen relative decreases in earning potential, we remain among the most affluent members of our society and, therefore, the world.

Although we believe ourselves to be generous, average Americans give away less than 1 percent of their income, or about $300 annually. According to pollster George Barna, evangelical Christians do significantly better, but average only about 4 percent, or $2,476 a year. Giving as a percentage among Americans, and specifically among Christians, has steadily dropped over the last fifty years, despite the fact that our relative earnings have markedly grown. American culture, particularly through the media, puts relentless pressure on Christian doctors to keep more of what they make, to acquire and accumulate, even if it means ignoring the needy or incurring debt. We've heard messages like: "You deserve more" and "Who says you can't have it all?" quite often. As a result, we've become convinced that we deserve the rewards of an ever-expanding American affluence. For physicians and dentists, the message seems to ring true because of our hard work and years of delayed gratification.

When Christians do give, it is generally not to meet the needs of the poor, but to support non-profit religious organizations. Among evangelicals, an average of 95 percent of their donations go to their churches. While it is true that churches pass along some of those funds to the poor, the percentage of "benevolence" has been declining, even as donations to churches have steadily grown. Many evangelical churches have elected to spend extensively, in some cases millions of dollars, on buildings, recreational facilities, and other programs that primarily serve their congregants, without corresponding increases in funding for missionary outreach or service to the needy. In many instances, our churches mirror our own personal spending patterns – more for us and less for the needy.

Among some conservatives, there exists a general suspicion of efforts to meet the physical needs of the poor. This impulse has been bolstered by the fact that some Christian denominations and organizations have stressed serving the poor while seemingly denying the importance of proclaiming Jesus and his gospel. Additionally, some Christians believe that many of the poor are not deserving of assistance, being responsible for their own lot through unwise or immoral choices. And lately, the church has been retreating from its historic role of serving the poor, expecting federal and local government agencies to meet those needs.

For all of those reasons (our lack of generosity as individuals and churches, our hesitancy to support charitable services that don't explicitly proclaim the gospel, our suspicion of the poor, and our mistaken reliance on the government) we have abandoned the clear teachings of the Scriptures and the Savior. We are like the rich man of Luke 16–dressed in fine clothes, living in luxuriously appointed homes, traveling in unnecessarily expensive vehicles. All the while, "at our gates" lie people like Lazarus, covered with sores and longing to eat what falls from our tables.

Peter Yok was only eleven years old when Muslim soldiers attacked his Christian village in southern Sudan. Like thousands of young Sudanese, Peter was permanently separated from his parents and other family members. After spending several years in a refugee camp in a neighboring African country, Peter was granted permission to immigrate to the United States.

On arriving he was given a few hundred dollars to pay for food and the rent on a sparse apartment in a declining section of town. Having received some instruction in English while in the refugee camp, Peter was able to secure low-wage employment in a factory that was accessible by bus. He was granted Medicaid health insurance for nine months. Apart from the emergency room at the nearby county hospital, there were no primary health providers near his apartment willing to accept his Medicaid insurance.

Across the globe and around the corner, we have the poor at our gates. While Americans enjoy an unrivaled standard of living, 2.8 billion people (nearly half of the world's population), live on less than two dollars a day. Here at home, 12 percent of Americans live at or below the established poverty level, the majority of those being women and children.

The collective hardship and suffering of so many people, particularly women and children, is so overwhelming that many of us have chosen to turn away. Our ability to do so is facilitated by the fact that we can live our lives without having much real contact with the poor. For some Christian physicians and dentists, our affluent suburbs, social organizations, educational institutions, and even our churches make it possible to largely avoid meaningful interaction with the needy, except in distant or token ways.

Such a world makes it easier to forget the needs of the poor and subsequently to accumulate more for the purposes of personal and family consumption. One generation of affluent Christians teaches the next generation, by virtue of the economic choices they make, to build prosperous and protected lives. Without careful consideration, we can unknowingly blend in comfortably with our self-directed culture. In that case, we neither honor God, nor help our needy neighbors.

The solution, of course, is simple to identify, but painful to implement. If we want to honor our King with a radical and growing obedience, we have to change our attitudes and actions regarding money. What we possess is

We are like the rich man of Luke 16—dressed in fine clothes, living in luxuriously appointed homes, traveling in unnecessarily expensive vehicles. All the while, "at our gates" lie people like Lazarus, covered with sores and longing to eat what falls from our tables.

If we're wise, we'll understand that we can generate great spiritual benefit for others and ourselves if we use the resources God has entrusted to us more for the furtherance of his Kingdom and less for our own safety and comfort. Jesus taught that we should live in such a way as to exceed the teachings of the Law and the Prophets, by the power of the Holy Spirit.

not ours, but belongs to the Master—all of it—as Jesus taught in the parable of the shrewd manager. It's not *our* salary, *our* bonus, *our* pension, *our* portfolio, *our* home, or even *our* family. If we're wise, we'll understand that we can generate great spiritual benefit for others and ourselves if we use the resources God has entrusted to us more for the furtherance of his kingdom and less for our own safety and comfort.

This has painfully practical applications:

- Where will we live?
- What will we drive?
- How shall we vacation?
- How much will we give...and to whom?
- How can we most strategically deploy the financial resources we have to honor Jesus and meet the needs of the poor?
- How can we manage what God has given us so that we are storing up true treasures in heaven?

There are no simple, black-and-white rules that can be applied to these questions, but the questions must be asked and answered prayerfully. Pastor and author John Piper states it this way:

> "...we must make sacrificial life choices rooted in the assurance that magnifying Christ through generosity and mercy is more satisfying than selfishness. If we walk away from risk to keep ourselves safe and solvent, we will waste our lives...if we look like our lives are devoted to getting and maintaining things, we will look like the world, and that will not make Christ look great."

Focus on Giving

Jesus taught that we should live in such a way as to exceed the teachings of the Law and the Prophets, by the power of the Holy Spirit. If Israel was instructed to be open-handed toward the needy, what should our stance be? Is 10 percent an adequate amount for Christian doctors to give away, or perhaps a starting point? What would happen if Christians began to recognize that the Law and the Prophets, the Apostles, and Jesus himself, put a high priority on generously, even sacrificially, giving to the needy?

If Christians increased their collective giving, only to the point of the tithe, there would be hundreds of millions of new dollars available to meet needs. Christian physicians and dentists must increasingly take risks in the name of love and generosity, having faith that God will meet their deepest needs far better than their empty materialistic culture can meet them. Perhaps there are some who would choose to sell superfluous assets and make those funds available for the purposes of generosity. Perhaps others might forego acquiring new possessions so that more resources can go to meeting material and spiritual needs. Who will model this lifestyle of generosity for the next generation of Christian physicians and dentists?

Whatever our percentage of giving, does it make sense to allocate the vast majority of our giving to institutions that largely service our needs and wants? Churches need and deserve financial support, but it is fair to ask whether they should receive such a large percentage of giving, while the poor are in such dire straits. If leaders in churches more fully recognized the biblical imperatives to give to the needy, there might be a reallocating of resources to better reflect a balance between generosity toward the needy and service to the congregation.

What if Christian physicians and dentists, often leaders in churches, began to make that case within their own congregations? Christian physicians and dentists must recognize that we have been given a great trust, a trust of both financial resources and influence. We have not always proven to be good stewards of that trust. We have the potential, however, to lead our families and our churches toward a lifestyle of biblical generosity.

GLEANINGS

On a personal level, is there a way that Christian doctors might apply, in a new and expansive way, the Old Testament principle of *the gleanings*? "When you harvest the grapes in your vineyard, do not go over the vines again. Leave what remains for the alien, the fatherless and the widow" (Deut. 24:21).

The principle was to leave some of the fruit of one's labor for the needy, rather than squeezing out every possible advantage. The edges of the fields, the olives that didn't fall with the first shaking of the trees, the grapes that the harvesters missed, all were to be left so that the needy might benefit. The command was accompanied by a promise: "When you are harvesting in your field and you overlook a sheaf, do not go back to get it. Leave it for the alien, the fatherless, and the widow, so that the LORD your God may bless you in all the work of your hands" (Deut. 24:19).

The gleanings of a Christian physician or dentist may be aspects of our work analogous to the edges of the field or the overlooked bunch of grapes. How can we apply this principle to our lives and practices? What might be the subsequent blessings from God? How might he further bless the work of our hands as we obey this principle?

Christian physicians and dentists must increasingly take risks in the name of love and generosity, having faith that God will meet their deepest needs far better than their empty materialistic culture can meet them.

*For some
it may mean
opening
their practice
to a limited
number of
uninsured
or poorly
insured
patients,
recognizing
that the
majority of
the medically
underserved
are poor
women
and children.*

Again, there cannot be across-the-board rules in the matter generosity. We can only consider the possibilities within the context of our own life and then, in faith and dependence on the Holy Spirit, look for ways to be sacrificially generous:

♦For some it may mean opening their practice to a limited number of uninsured or poorly insured patients, recognizing that the majority of the medically underserved are poor women and children. Many of these patients might not appear obviously needy, as was the case with Marilyn Ziegler (this chapter's opening story). From a purely economic perspective, caring for such patients might seem unwise, but those who take such a risk can rely on God's promise that he will "bless you in all the work of your hands."

♦God may lead some to write off past or present charges for patients who are hard-pressed to pay.

♦The principle of gleanings for some may mean committing their vacation or work time to serving the medical or dental needs of the poor in the developing world or among the needy in the US. There are numerous opportunities to pursue these options through CMDA.

♦Many Christian physicians and dentists have acquired business skills that could be employed in assisting a new or expanded ministry outreach to the poor. Christian community health centers are far more likely to succeed if they have strong medical or dental leadership.

♦Some of us have learned to influence organizations and institutions through our leadership and communication skills. Physicians and dentists, because of their prestige, have been successful at lobbying hospitals and government to advance their professional and financial agendas. There are some among us whose gleanings lie in their ability to influence medical groups, universities, medical societies, or government agencies on behalf of the poor. If we spend significant amounts of money to insure protection from government intrusion or fair payment for services rendered, might we exert similar pressure on behalf of those with little or no influence? Christians have an honorable record of lobbying on behalf of the unborn; might we expand our vision to include protecting other vulnerable members of our society? Would not such intercession on behalf of the poor honor our King and demonstrate to the world that God and his people love "the least of these"?

Many CMDA members have found creative ways to honor our King through their giving and gleanings. Here are ten suggestions:

1. *Simplify your lifestyle.* Remove from your life excess possessions or expenditures that may distract you or blind you to those in great need.
2. *Increase your overall giving* to at least a tithe.
3. *Encourage your church* to use more of its resources in demonstrating God's concern for the poor.
4. *Open your practice* to a limited number of uninsured patients. Consider the tithe here as well.
5. *Develop a team* of physician and dentist consultants who are willing to help you with uninsured patients.
6. *With your hospital, develop a plan* for economic screening and mutual charity care for the poor
7. *Be willing to risk loss of income and loss of time* in order to follow God's commands toward the poor.
8. *Volunteer one night a month* at a health care facility for the poor.
9. *Work politically for adequate healthcare for the poor*, even if it threatens your income.
10. *Ask God if he wishes you to work full-time in healthcare for the poor*.

Dr. Luke has much to teach us about our responsibility to the poor. Let us accept his diagnosis and proceed with the prescription he offers. The therapeutic plan begins with our honest recognition that God's concern for the poor is not a small thing, but rather occupies a prominent place in his heart, his kingdom, and the Scriptures. The subject has not received the attention or emphasis from Christians that it deserves.

According to the Bible, those who enrich themselves and ignore the poor are in grave spiritual danger, even if they think themselves believers. Doing good for others is not a means to salvation; we are saved because God in his mercy chooses to save us, through faith, by the costly sacrifice of his Son. Nonetheless, those who are truly recipients of God's gracious salvation will demonstrate their faith by a radical and growing obedience to the teachings of Jesus and the Apostles. We are to emulate a shrewd manager who uses his master's possessions to benefit himself. May Christian physicians and dentists have the courage and faith to use all that God has entrusted to us for his glory and the benefit of others, knowing that we are building up eternal treasures for ourselves in heaven. May we have the courage and faith to recognize that we who are abundantly blessed must change our patterns of consumption in order to redirect resources to the needy. May we make

Would not such intercession on behalf of the poor honor our King and demonstrate to the world that God and his people love "the least of these"?

*May we
have the
courage and
faith to
recognize
that we
who are
abundantly
blessed
must
change our
patterns of
consumption,
in order to
redirect
resources
to the needy.*

personal and organizational choices that better reflect God's concern for the poor, always looking for ways that we can fulfill these responsibilities in new and expansive ways in accordance with our great King's new kingdom. Such faith-driven obedience will honor God, help the needy, and demonstrate to the world what and whom we truly love.

THREE QUESTIONS TO ASK YOURSELF

1. How much attention have I given to the biblical commands to serve the poor directly?
2. What percentage of my giving goes to meeting the needs of the poor?
3. What aspect of my practice could be considered gleanings for the needy?

THREE ACTIONS TO CONSIDER

1. Read through the gospel of Luke, purposefully looking for teachings about the poor.
2. Give at or above the tithe, with a significant amount going directly to meeting the needs of the poor.
3. Identify and enlarge your gleanings.

PRAYER

Lord Jesus, you are the richest person in the universe, having created everything, yet, in taking on humanity you chose to become poor. I confess that I have not rightly reflected your concern for the poor, but have been quick to spend your resources on my own comfort and safety. Please teach me to love you more than I love your gracious gifts. Teach me to demonstrate my growing trust in you by a radical generosity toward the poor.

—Amen

CHAPTER 7

The Practice of Compassion

*H*olly was admitted to the hospital for a seizure disorder that developed when her breast cancer found its way into her spinal fluid. She remained confused for a number of days, but she smiled each time she spotted me beside her bed. One morning after I had examined her, her sister stepped out of the room with me and described Holly's home life to me. Holly's husband was very cold emotionally and was often verbally abusive to her in spite of her ongoing physical suffering.

"It's different when she comes to see you, Dr. Weir. When I pick her up to bring her for an appointment, she beams and says, 'I get my hug today.'"

There was very little that I could do for Holly in the way of therapy against her cancer. At the best, all the tricks in my bag to attack carcinomatous meningitis would hold back her disease for but a few months.

What then was it that I offered as her doctor that made my work so meaningful to her?

–Al Weir, M.D.

As doctors we sometimes lose sight of the legitimate goals of our work for our patients. Sometimes we focus on disease, when God has placed us here to focus on people. There are four worthwhile goals of our work as doctors:

1. We should always work to prevent illness or its complications in our patients;
2. Cure the illnesses that cause suffering in our patients if at all possible;
3. Sometimes cure is not possible, as is the case with many cancers, diabetes, and coronary artery disease. In these situations, a worthwhile goal is to help our patients live as long as possible in spite of their illnesses;

Our responsibility in caring for patients who suffer lies within a two-fold mission we need to pursue; specifically, to reduce suffering and to offer hope and value.

4. No matter which of the first three goals is operative, and even if none of them is achievable, the fourth legitimate goal for medical and dental practitioners is to help all of our patients experience the best quality of life possible.

The fourth goal is the subject of this chapter. Our responsibility as caregivers goes far beyond easing pain. It encompasses the emotional, physical, and spiritual well-being of those who come to us for help. How can we do this well? How can we actually care for our patients while we are attempting to fight their disease? How can we practice compassion? Our responsibility in caring for patients who suffer lies within a two-fold mission we need to pursue; specifically, to reduce suffering and to offer hope and value.

REDUCE SUFFERING

Most doctors are trained to reduce the suffering of their patients. We must keep this goal in mind even as we fight disease so we don't add more suffering by our treatment than the illness causes by its presence. I'm reminded of the patient who underwent anesthesia for a circumcision and woke up without a penis. His urologist had discovered a penile cancer while the patient was asleep and had taken care of it then and there. A year later the patient was still struggling with the shock of his discovery on awakening from anesthesia. The treatment was necessary and the patient is cured of his disease; the doctor handled that part of his responsibility well. Nevertheless, the patient suffered emotionally because the cure came about without proper discussion and compassion prior to the amputation.

We can reduce the suffering of our patients by keeping six things in mind:

1. Do the Science Well

This is what our patients come to us for. They expect us to be well trained, skilled, and up-to-date with the scientific management of their problem. Very little else we do matters if we fail them at the point of competence. We reduce our patients' suffering best if we can work with God to cure their diseases. However, we have an even greater responsibility to reduce suffering if we deal with an illness that we cannot eradicate. How well we manage the blood sugar of a diabetic matters when we look ahead to the long-term complications of that disease. How well we manage periodontal disease impacts our patient's long-term oral suffering. Our scientific competence in managing the diseases of our patients is more likely to reduce their suffering than any other factor in their care.

Does our scientific competence count when the disease itself is not the target? Of course it does. How well we do pain management matters to a patient with metastatic breast cancer to the bone. How well we handle constipation may be the most important way we can reduce the suffering of patients on pain medicine. How adept we are in managing disorientation and delirium matters in the suffering of our Alzheimer's patients. Whether we are attacking the disease itself or dealing with parallel symptoms, our competence in the science of our patients' illnesses is critical. Our scientific abilities in reducing the suffering of our patients come from study, training, and hard work, all of which require our most valuable personal commodity: time. We must take the time and do the work necessary to be the best scientific doctors we can be if we wish to be part of God's method of reducing the suffering of our patients.

Sometimes our patients need our ear more than they need our medicine.

2. Listen

Do we take the time to listen to our patients? Sometimes they need our ear more than they need our medicine. How often have you had an experience similar to the following?

I walked into the examining room to find a patient who had been added to my schedule. Her history was one of breast cancer with a relatively low risk for recurrence. In the middle of my incredibly busy schedule making life and death decisions for other patients with active cancer, this patient began relating in prolonged detail a problem with her ears that was clearly benign. I forced myself to sit still for the duration of her description, glued to the chair by her level of anxiety. After a brief examination, I explained to her that the discomfort she felt in her right ear was related to a viral illness causing pressure on her eustachian tube. At that point she broke down and cried. "My sister died when her cancer spread to her brain," she said. "I thought that was happening to me and I haven't slept in three nights. Thank you, doctor." In spite of all the major cancer-related decisions I made the rest of the day, I probably relieved more suffering by listening during those twenty minutes than I did in the next twenty patients I saw.

—Al Weir, M.D.

Most doctors would choose to take the time to listen to our patients if our lives were not so fast-paced and hectic. One of the chief reasons patients migrate to alternative health practitioners is that those providers listen to their patients, and that relieves suffering. Can we do a better job than we now do? There are three changes many of us need to make in order to listen better: (1) Choose to see listening as an instrument of healing instead of

Remember that it is not only what we say, but how we say it that may matter most to our patients.

as a problem of time; (2) Refuse to think of life outside the room where we are sitting with our patients; (3) Schedule fewer patients so we can give a listening ear to those who need it.

3. Communicate

Outside of Paul's room I had a disagreement with his wife about the best location for his terminal care. I had fought his cancer battle with him for over a year, producing better than expected results. I loved him but his long struggle was now nearly over. I wanted him in a facility where I could still help manage his quality of life issues. His wife had chosen one where I could not be involved. She would not budge from her decision. I finally quit trying to change her mind, with the comment, "I'll take care of it." Then I turned away quickly to finish my rounds. The next day the wife's brother told me how I had hurt her feelings by being so abrupt, and that I needed to mend the relationship.

–Al Weir, M.D.

This doctor had a problem with communication, an arena in which we can develop skills that will enhance our ability to relieve the suffering of our patients. Here are some suggestions:

•Remember that it is not only what we say, but how we say it that may matter most to our patients. Body language often says more than words. Sit down. Face patients fully for your entire encounter without one foot lined up with the door. At some point, close the chart, look into their eyes and fold your hands. Each of these steps tells patients that you are committed to them as persons. They are then much more likely to hear your words and follow your suggestions.

•Provide more than data with your words. If our patients needed only information in order to manage their illnesses, the Internet would provide more than we could hope to provide. It is our interpretation of this information for them that transforms data into understanding and makes our communication useful to them. Here are some tips: Talk normally, using a language as close to theirs as possible. Your patients think with their own language. Get there if you can. Remember that patients often do not hear what you think you are telling them. Say what you mean in two or three different ways, if necessary, to help them understand. Two very helpful tools to enhance new patients' understanding are to provide them written information about their illness and to tape discussions with them so they can listen again at home when the shock of the visit has worn off.

•Whenever bad news is given, during the same visit present your patients with reasonable goals of therapy and a plan to reach those goals. For example, you might say, "We may not be able to cure your cancer, but we can control it for a number of years and here's how we might go about doing that."

•Use humor when appropriate. Always look for an avenue to bring a smile into their lives. Even seriously ill patients feel better when they laugh.

An elderly redhead once entered my office after a mastectomy. She bounced in and offered, "Doctor, you have got to feel my new artificial breast." I protested, but she insisted until I pressed my hand against it. She squealed and said, "Doctor, you've got the wrong one!" Then she laughed out loud as I blushed. "Just kidding," she said. And then we both laughed.

—Al Weir, M.D.

It is not always easy to help a patient laugh in the face of a serious illness. If we do it poorly, we may belittle their suffering; but if we can make them laugh in spite of their illness, there are few things that can reduce their suffering more for the moment.

•After the data, after you've listed the options of therapy, after they've had time to think, help guide them toward a decision. For example, you might say, "It's your decision, but if you were my sister, I would suggest you do it this way." Even though patient autonomy is central in American medicine, doctors should not let go of their responsibilities as counselors.

4. Deal with their Emotions

They flew her in from Pensacola. I thought they had brought her home to die. A brain tumor had left her staring into space and unable to speak. I stood outside the room and told her son that she would not recover. I was as compassionate as I knew how to be. I told him that he was in charge, but, if she were my mother, I would let her die without placing her on a ventilator or putting her through a lot of difficult tests. I thought he understood, but by the time I reached the office, the son had called, boiling mad, requesting another doctor because I wanted to let his mother die.

—Al Weir, M.D.

Emotions are a natural part of our lives, put there for value. They are also a natural part of dealing with pain. The emotion experienced by the

Always look for an avenue to bring a smile into their lives. Even seriously ill patients feel better when they laugh.

If their emotions cause them to suffer, then we need to face that suffering and deal with it for their own good.

patient's son in this case—anger—is natural when patients suffer from painful or debilitating illness, and the anger they feel can cause them more suffering than the illness itself. Our job in healthcare is to relieve the suffering of our patients. If their emotions cause them to suffer, then we need to face that suffering and deal with it for their own good. Anger is a particularly harmful emotion. If we can reduce anger, we succeed in our task to reduce suffering. The same would be true of despair or fear. Dr. David Allen, in a talk to Christian doctors, described five steps we can take to help our patients reduce their pain by reducing their anger:

1. Help them **recognize** their anger. Sometimes patients are miserable and irritable and don't realize that their misery is due to anger. Just as the first step in overcoming alcoholism is recognizing you are an alcoholic, the first step in overcoming anger is realizing you are angry.

2. Help them **rationalize** their anger. Sometimes patients are angry by reflex from their pain and have never thought through their situation to see if their anger is reasonable. Walking a patient through the process that led to their anger may point out some misunderstanding or provide a "new understanding" that would help the anger dissipate.

3. Help them **relate** their anger. Anger grows when it is held close to the heart. We need to encourage our patients to discuss their anger with those who have caused it or those who have been injured by it. If anger is felt toward God, our patients should continue to discuss it with him and not turn silent toward their Creator.

4. Help them **relinquish** their rights. As humans, we feel we have the right to health and happiness. Christians relinquish these rights and hand them over to the Father. Sometimes illness causes us to take back those rights from the him. If our patients are Christians, we can lovingly encourage them to remember Col. 3:3: "For you have died and your life is hid with Christ in God" (RSV).

5. Help them **release** their anger. Anger, like sin, can destroy our relationship with those we love and with God. Eventually, our patients need to lay their anger at the foot of the cross, where they have placed their sin, and let the blood of the Lamb cleanse it from their lives.

Just as we can help our patients deal with their anger, we need to evaluate all of their emotional suffering and develop the skills to help them relieve that suffering. Often with emotional suffering, we need to enlist help from other professionals, counselors, family, or friends.

5. Focus on the Family

Some time ago, I cared for a man with cancer who was also suffering from Alzheimer's. The net result was that all worthwhile communication came from the family. One particular brother who was staying with the patient was obnoxious. He would often make unreasonable demands and consistently focus on irrelevant details in his brother's care. I began spending less and less time in the patient's room. I became shorter and shorter with my answers to the family's questions, considering them annoying rather than helpful to my patient's care, until I realized what I was doing.

—Al Weir, M.D.

Sometimes it is tempting to think: *I've got enough to do just to take care of my patients; the family members will have to take care of themselves.* If we act on those thoughts, we fail in one of our responsibilities as Christian doctors; specifically, to care for our patients' families as we care for our patients.

The fact is, our patient's quality of life is often dependent on the family. The family may be necessary to help with healthcare management in areas such as diet, injections, transportation, and surveillance for symptoms. In addition to technical assistance, patients' families provide the emotional environment within which patients live with their illnesses. Our patients suffer less within an environment of peace, love, and gentleness than within one of bitterness, confusion, and hostility. The way we deal with the family directly impacts the suffering of our patients.

Beyond this, as persons of compassion, we need to remember that the family members of our patients are suffering human beings as well. Sometimes the pain—especially the emotional suffering—is greater when it is your loved one who suffers than when the suffering is your own. As Christian doctors, we should take on the responsibility of reducing the suffering of our patients' families whenever this is possible.

6. Encourage Community

Helen was an artist who had painted two beautiful oil paintings for my office and home. She had colon cancer and would not live long with her disease. One day she came in beaming about her experience in our treatment room. "We have so much fun in there; we don't need another support group," she said. "We laugh;

One of our responsibilities as Christian doctors is to care for our patients' families as we care for our patients.

we cry; we hug; we exchange tough times; and, we exchange recipes. I always leave there feeling I've been lifted up."

—Al Weir, M.D.

One of the major causes of suffering for some patients is isolation. The more serious their illness is, the more likely they will fall outside of normality and be different. Sometimes this leads them to withdraw from their previous activities and relationships. They become lonely and they suffer for it.

To the best of our ability as doctors, any help we can provide in moving our isolated patients back into community will reduce their suffering. In the time we spend with our patients, we need to discover their normal channels of activity and whether they have isolated themselves unnecessarily from those activities because of their illness. Then we should encourage them to resume the old activities or initiate new ones to protect them from the pain of isolation. We particularly need to be committed to getting our patients into a church community where people of faith can offer them hope and love.

Whether they admit it or not, our patients suffer greatly if they are left alone with their illness. We as Christian doctors should take the time to know our patients well enough to be aware of these social connections. Then through encouragement, referral, consultation, or social service, we should try to make sure our patients are buffered from their pain by people who care about them.

ADD VALUE AND HOPE

As Christian doctors, we can help reduce the suffering of our patients. That's what the world is crying for. But if all we can do is reduce suffering, life still may not be worth living for our patients. Can we provide something for our patients beyond a reduction in their suffering? Certainly. Christian doctors have a responsibility, as do all Christians, to help add value and hope to their patients' lives. Doctors, more than most people, have the skills and opportunity to do so. What does it mean to add value and hope to our patients' lives?

Bernie is a friend of mine. One day while we were seated around his fireplace on a cold winter's eve, he told us about his mom. When Bernie was young, he was poor and his mother was single. They were so poor that they could not even afford to fix his eyeglasses and Bernie had to use a safety pin to hold them together. One day, at Grahamwood Elementary School, it began to snow. The teachers were

To the best of our ability as doctors, any help we can provide in moving our isolated patients back into community will reduce their suffering.

merciful and let all the kids out for awhile to play. Bernie was a dutiful son and placed his glasses carefully in his pocket before he went out into the snow. When the recess was over, Bernie unzipped his coat and reached for his glasses but they were gone. Bernie realized that his mother would be upset and told his teacher, who let all the kids go back out onto the playground to search for Bernie's glasses. The snow continued to fall and the glasses could not be found. When school was over, Bernie walked home to face his mother whom he knew would be disappointed in him. After hearing Bernie's story, rather than yelling at him, Bernie's mother took him by the hand and walked him back to school. When they arrived at the playground, she asked Bernie to show her where he had lost his glasses. Bernie, in exasperation, waved his hand over the entire field and shouted, "We went everywhere!" Bernie's mother paused and prayed, then trudged across the snow covered field. Bernie saw her lean over, brush away a layer of snow, and pick up his glasses. She handed Bernie his glasses and they walked home together.

–Al Weir, M.D.

If we treat the diseases of our patients, and do nothing more, we may well only brush away the snow that covers a life lying broken on the frozen earth. We can do more. We can pick up the glasses of hope and value that have lain beneath the snow and hand them back to our patients so they can see again a world worth living in. In fact, as Christian doctors, we may be able to help them see value and hope greater than they have ever seen before.

Adjusting their Focus

One of the problems with pain and suffering is that it forces patients to focus on themselves. Biologically, that makes sense, because we all need to focus on our problems in order to correct them. Medically, that's why our patients come to us, so we can focus on their problems and try to fix them. One problem of self-focus, however, is that it can lead patients to let go of life beyond their physical distress, the part of life that contains much of their hope and value. Doctors can help bring back that hope and value if we help our patients adjust their focus.

Peggy had lung cancer, and little time to live. As she sat before me that day, I accidentally stumbled onto the question, "Can you tell me something good that's happened to you since I saw you last?" Her eyes lit up and she answered, "Oh, yes! My kids were over this weekend and we had the greatest time." Peggy related how they had actually had fun with each other dividing up things in the house that would be part of their inheritance. She told me how one of her grandchildren had asked her, "What happened to your hair?" When she explained about the chemotherapy, the child told her, "If you saved it, you can make it wet, then pat it

If we treat the diseases of our patients, and do nothing more, we may well only brush away the snow that covers a life lying broken on the frozen earth.

on your head and it will stick."

Peggy laughed at these memories and her day was better.

—Al Weir, M.D.

Simple questions like the one asked above can help patients focus away from their illness and toward the people they love. A moment of hopelessness can be transformed into a moment of value. With our knowledge of their lives outside their illness, doctors can make statements, ask questions, and point out possibilities that will help them focus on the continued value of life outside their difficulties. But to where can we point them that they will not see their pain?

•We can point them toward good memories. "I hear you like golfing," we might say. "What's the best course you ever played?" or "I passed by your business yesterday. What was it like getting that business going?" or "Do you think it was as tough playing football back then as it is now?" Questions like these are more than small talk. They can be instruments in our hands to relieve suffering by helping patients in pain focus on better times.

•We can point them toward good relationships. "How is your daughter doing? I heard she won an award for teaching." or "Do you and your wife still play tennis together?" The best of life is bound up in relationships. With illnesses, patients often let go of the hands that gave them meaning in life. We can help them rebuild those relationships.

•We can point them toward good events. "Are you coming to the park for the sunset symphony?" or "Have you got a vacation planned this summer?" or "Have you been to visit your daughter and grandson lately?" An event is a goal and goals require living to get to, not just suffering to go through.

•We can point them toward the Father. "This certainly is a difficult problem. I think I can help you, but we need all the help we can get. Do you mind if I pray with you about this?" or "I know this illness has been very difficult for you. How are you holding up emotionally? How are you holding up spiritually?"

As doctors, we must ignore the fact that questions and statements like these add time to our patient encounters. They are no different from the surgeon's scalpel or the prescription pad in treating our patients as human beings who suffer. They are instruments that must be used if we wish to relieve suffering by adjusting the focus of our patients away from their pain so that value and hope can return to their lives.

Stimulate a Thankful Heart

I can remember Donna well—ex-missionary, church hostess, good friend. She suffered as much from cancer as anyone I have seen. Rarely do I fail to control cancer pain to a bearable level, but with her I could not; and yet she rarely complained and was never bitter. On her last night of life she sat up in the bed and said, "Alright, alright. Thank you, Jesus." Her niece asked her what she was thanking Jesus for and Donna answered, "For all he has done for me. It's almost over." She then lay back and slept peacefully through the night until she slipped into heaven.

The poorest people I have known were the African villagers from Sanubi. I will never forget the sweltering Nigerian morning when I thought the church service was over, but discovered that it had just begun. The church members began gathering at the back of the church in small groups. I watched as each group marched down to the front of the church, singing as they danced, and laying money on the table. Group after group sang and carried their thanksgiving offerings to the altar. Church members were not satisfied to join one group; they would repeat their thanksgiving journey in multiple groups, laying money down each time. These were the poorest people I've ever known and, at that moment, some of the happiest, giving money to the God who had helped them through their year. One of their songs went like this:

> *"What will I render unto my God?*
> *What will I render unto my Savior?*
> *I will give all my life to him.*
> *I will give all my life to him."*

—Al Weir, M.D.

A thankful spirit is not something you can forcibly put on, like a suit of clothes when you want to get dressed. A thankful heart comes from being aware of your blessings. Our job as doctors, therefore, is to help patients become aware of their blessings. "How many years have you been married to that sweet wife of yours?" we might ask. "Not many men get that kind of woman to take care of them." Or, "So your daughter's grown and out on her own? It's a blessing when we can get our children that far." Or, "Man, isn't it great we have a God we can turn to in tough times!"

Questions that help our patients adjust their focus are instruments that must be used if we wish to relieve their suffering and help value and hope return to their lives.

If we understand that our mission to relieve suffering also includes helping patients develop a thankful heart, then we can regularly point them to areas of blessing in their lives.

If we are focused, if we have taken the time to get to know our patients, if we understand that our mission to relieve suffering also includes helping patients develop a thankful heart, then we can regularly point them to areas of blessing in their lives–blessings from their past, blessings coming to them in the future, blessings from relationships, blessings from God's presence, and blessings from our guaranteed victory in heaven. It takes time; it takes caring; it takes knowing who our patients are; it takes commitment to transform a bitter heart into a thankful one, slowly, and with God's Spirit doing most of the work.

Make Life Real Again

One thing that sometimes happens to our patients with serious illness is the loss of feeling normal. They can think: *Because of this problem I'm not like other folks anymore.* Until they are ill, some patients don't realize that being normal sometimes involves having serious problems; so, when trouble comes, they feel separated from real life and suffer on the outside of humanity's huddle.

We can help bring people who suffer back into the bounds of real human experience, and thus diminish their suffering of isolation by touching them and connecting them with others who have goals to accomplish and a sense of mission in life:

- ◆Real people laugh
- ◆Real people fellowship
- ◆Real people touch
- ◆Real people have goals to accomplish and a mission to live

We have already mentioned the importance of laughter and fellowship; what about touch? As doctors, we should purposely use touch as part of our ministry to suffering people. Jesus almost always touched those he healed. Touch demonstrates commitment. Touch reinforces personal worth. Touch relieves isolation.

I remember well the fingerless leper in Nigeria, living in a colony of lepers, his face scarred with the disease. I held back my hand for a moment, until I realized that it was all I had of value to give. When I shook that diseased hand, he smiled a crooked smile and suffered less that day. A handshake or a touch on the shoulder may relieve more pain than any injection of morphine.

–Al Weir, M.D.

One of the strongest sources of value is a sense of mission: the understanding that we are reaching for a goal and accomplishing something worthwhile in our lives. Sometimes our patients, because of their illness, have lost that sense of mission.

Mission is important to our patients for a number of reason. Mission provides a goal to accomplish. Mission provides a focus away from their troubles. Mission provides a sense of self-worth. Mission is what normal people do, so mission provides a connection with the living. And, mission is more than all that. Mission is what God plans for us no matter what our health circumstances. Mission lets us take part in God's work in this world. The happiest patients we know are those who look beyond themselves toward helping others.

Victor Frankl was a psychiatrist who was imprisoned by the Nazi's at Auschwitz during the Holocaust. According to Frankl, only one in twenty-eight of his fellow prisoners survived their stay at Auschwitz. Out of that experience came Frankl's great work entitled *Man's Search for Meaning*. Dr. Frankl's suffering in Auschwitz was as great or greater than the suffering experienced by most patients.

In reflecting on that terrible suffering, Dr. Frankl wrote, "If there is a meaning in life at all, there must be a meaning in suffering." He wasn't talking of philosophical meaning, but of very practical meaning that benefited one's self or one's neighbors. He continued, "We had to learn ourselves and furthermore, we had to teach the despairing men, that it did not really matter what we expected from life, but rather what life expected from us."

Our happiest patients are those who, through their suffering, have searched to find what life expects from them. From within their own suffering they have looked beyond themselves to seek out ways to serve those around them, in all kinds of ways.

The happiest patients we know are those who look beyond themselves toward helping others.

One patient I know cuts his neighbor's grass and weeds his flower bed. Another makes beautiful cards with her personal artwork, and then sends them to those who need encouragement. Myra Max has lymphoma and over the years has printed thousands of inspirational cards entitled "What Cancer Can't Do." Many patients have taken these cards and gained hope for their lives. One might try to say that some patients are just nobler than others, while some have all they can do just to lick their own wounds. I don't believe that's true. It is not because they are noble that some serve others. It is in serving others that those who suffer become noble and find joy in the process.

–Al Weir, M.D.

*It is not
because
they are
noble that
some serve
others.
It is in
serving
others that
those
who suffer
become
noble
and find
joy in
the process.*

One's sense of mission can be developed even when one doesn't feel like it. We as doctors, having completed our medical care in visits with our patients, can encourage their service to God and others. For example, we might say, "John, I'm glad your diabetes is coming under control. You've worked hard at it. God has given you new strength. Make sure you are using it well. Have you ever thought about volunteering to help other people who are sick?"

The words we use will be different for every patient, but somehow we need to help our patients reestablish mission in their lives. They will not only feel their pain less, they will add value to their lives that may even make their illness worthwhile. It may even have eternal results, as this story illustrates:

My nurse, Melanie, once told me: "My father had cancer and was a patient here before you came. Near the end of his life he had lost a leg to cancer, was weak and in pain, but he wanted to return to Guyana on a mission trip. He had been there many times before. We all tried to discourage him, but he insisted and went. It was a difficult trip for him and soon after his return, he died.

"But that's not the end of the story. This past Christmas a friend of mine came to visit me. She had moved to a small town in Arkansas and told me of a women's Bible study group she was part of. She told me that one day they were introducing themselves and a girl with a strange accent said, 'I'm from Guyana. I've only been a Christian for a short time. Missionaries used to come from the United States and my parents were saved long ago, but it didn't seem that important to me.

'Then one day, this missionary came, weak and wasted and limping so badly that he could hardly climb up the hill. When I saw him there, I listened. If that man had come in that condition to tell me about Jesus, I knew it must be important. That time I listened and became a Christian.'"

—Al Weir, M.D.

Seek Spiritual Dimensions

As Christian doctors, we understand that each of our patients is created for a relationship with their Father in heaven. Many don't have that relationship and others have let it diminish with the worries of life. Whatever we do for our patients medically, they all have life remaining that is nearly empty without God and they all will someday knock on the door to eternity. We must not doubt our responsibility as Christian doctors to encourage them toward a right relationship with God through Jesus, because the following are true:

•All of our patients need a different concept of time—death is not the end.

•All of our patients need a different concept of reality—life is more than we can touch.

•All of our patients need a different concept of value—that which is most dear in this life doesn't have to vanish.

•All of our patients need a relationship with the Father. It is in this relationship that our patients will find peace, purpose, power to overcome, the presence of God in all circumstances, and the promise that with Christ life goes on forever after death.

How do we help bring our patients to the feet of the Father? Another chapter deals with this in more detail, but here are a few steps to follow:

•Prepare the soil early with a spiritual history or in opening discussions as they establish themselves as new patients.

•Cultivate with faith flags—brief comments or statements that make your patients aware of your faith. These may be cards and signs in your office, but also must be words that point to God. "It was God who made you better. I just work for him."

•Pray with your patients when they give permission. Pray for your patients—always and regularly.

•Trust God with the harvest and be ready if he asks you to share the path to salvation.

Truly caring for our patients involves both the relief of suffering and the rekindling of hope and value in their lives. We fulfill these roles with actions that range from lancing a boil to introducing them to God. Christian doctors, of all people, have been blessed to be handed such a rewarding mission for our lives.

THREE QUESTIONS TO ASK YOURSELF

1. What questions can I easily ask some of my patients in order to help them focus on others?

2. What changes must I make in order to have the time I need to listen to and communicate with my patients?

3. Do I pray for my patients regularly?

THREE ACTIONS TO CONSIDER

1. This week, encourage one patient toward service to God or others.

2. One day in the office this week, make a point to touch each patient you encounter.

We must not doubt our responsibility as Christian doctors to encourage patients toward a right relationship with God through Jesus.

3. This week, ask the family members accompanying your patients how they are doing and whether you can help them in any way.

PRAYER

Dear Father,
What an awesome privilege you have given me to ease the suffering of people you love and to bring value and hope into their lives. Help me do this like Jesus did. If you can find ways for me to slow down and do it better, please show me. If not, teach me to do it fast. Let me not waste this mission you have handed me. Let your Spirit accomplish your redemptive purpose for my patients when I fail.

—Amen

CHAPTER 8

Missions

During the summer of 1977, we lived in Southern California and life was good. I had become the residency director of one of the most respected, oldest, and largest family practice programs in the United States. My academic appointment was with the UCLA School of Medicine, our affiliated medical school, and it looked like my career was on the fast track.

I loved teaching the Sunday school class many of the principles I had learned from Dr. Francis Schaeffer when we had studied with him at L'Abri in Huemoz, Switzerland, a few years earlier. My wife Jan loved her involvement in the young women's group.

We had a wonderful house with a pool that our kids lived in and a view that looked out over the San Bernardino Mountains. We enjoyed entertaining our Sunday school class and other groups from the church. We also had the residents from the training program over and saw it as an opportunity for ministry.

My father, who was a retired miller and small businessman from the Midwest thought it was particularly amazing to be able to swim in the heated pool and look up to the snow on the mountains. Our families would come out to visit and we delighted in showing them the Southern California attractions. Our children loved it all. Life was rich and fulfilling.

Then, while I was praying about what subject to teach next in Sunday school class, I heard a still, small voice within: "You are going to be making a change." That's all it was. My response was, "Not really. Why would I want to change this life – for what?" But again it would come in prayer, "You are going to be making a change."

And as I tried to pray for clarification or elaboration, that was all I got.

So I shared with Jan, "I feel like we are going to be making a change."

She replied, "If you are going somewhere else, you are going without me. I love my church, my Bible study group, my house, and living here."

God has given all Christians a universal mission to work with him as Lord to redeem the world.

I let it go, knowing that if what I was hearing was true, God would have to change her heart and mine.

That fall, I saw in a Christian magazine that a Christian university was going to start a medical school and was looking for faculty. I laughed and told Jan about it – what a crazy idea it was and how difficult it would be to succeed. I threw the magazine away and forgot about it until the next time I was praying about God's next direction in my life. Then the still small voice whispered, "I want you to go to Tulsa, be a part of that medical school and train Christian physicians."

My response was, "But God, I don't want to leave here and go to Tulsa." Yet each time I prayed, I heard the same message from the God who had fashioned the work for my life even before I was born (Eph. 2:10). I finally wrote a letter of "inquiry" and worded it in such a way that the university should not have been interested in me. Then I explained to God that I had done my part.

There followed a chain of events that ultimately led my wife and me to visit Tulsa. During that process, God provided a series of extraordinary confirmations. Had he not done so, I suspect we would have never left Southern California.

During our visit to Tulsa, we sensed a commitment to excellence and a real commitment to God's call by the future faculty and staff who were coming, many with extraordinary stories of how God had led them. We were impressed by the university's college students and wondered if the medical students (should they get the medical school approved) would be as bright, ministry-oriented, and spiritually attuned. We were assured they would be.

Having heard no new pronouncement from my wife about leaving Southern California, I asked her on the flight back what she thought.

There was a long and pregnant silence before she said, "I don't know what the big deal is all about; of course we will be going to Tulsa."

My heart leapt at that confirmation – we were off on a great adventure of faith. More extraordinary things continued to confirm our move as we went. It often seemed like the missionary stories we had heard about God's provision.

–John Crouch, M.D.

UNDERSTANDING OUR MISSION

God has given all Christians a universal mission to work with him as Lord to redeem the world:

All authority in heaven and on earth has been given to me. Go therefore and make disciples of all nations, baptizing them in the name of the Father and of the Son and of the Holy Spirit, teaching them to observe all that I have commanded you; and lo, I am with you always, to the close of the age (Matt. 28:18-20, RSV).

Once we have accepted Christ as Lord, we come under this command and this universal mission as part of our lives.

God has also created each of us with an individual mission for our lives. Each of us must seek that mission and live it out if our lives are to be fulfilled:

> For we are his workmanship, created in Christ Jesus for good works, which God prepared beforehand, that we should walk in them (Eph. 2:10, RSV).

God has a special plan for each of our lives. We must long for it, seek it, and carry it out to its completion. One minister put it this way, "I've got my own spiritual DNA."

God may call us out from our everyday life of mission to special missions that may be short-term or lifelong. Such missions may require a disruption of our routine lives in order to accomplish his special purpose:

> For if you keep silence at such a time as this, relief and deliverance will rise for the Jews from another quarter, but you and your father's house will perish. And who knows whether you have not come to the kingdom for such a time as this? (Esther 4:14, RSV).

Many doctors can remember a night by a soda machine, a campfire service, a tap on the shoulder, or a cry from the pulpit that was God's way of calling them to some special work that changed their life's routine for God's purpose.

Any missions endeavor to which God calls us may be a large or a small part of the life mission for which he created us. Only God knows how the whole plan fits together. Oswald Chambers' greatest legacy for the kingdom was not his mission to North Africa during the first World War, but the sermons his wife collected into the book My *Utmost for His Highest* after his death in North Africa.

Take a moment to answer these questions:

- Do I understand the differences between these biblical concepts related to mission?
- Where do I stand in terms of my sense of calling to universal mission as a Christian doctor?
- Where do I stand as an individual for whom God has a special purpose in life?
- Is God calling me into special missions service at this time of my life?

Any missions God calls us to may be a large or a small part of the life mission for which he created us. Only God knows how the whole plan fits together.

Then I felt God ask me, "What is in your hand? Where is your rod? What are the tools of your trade?" My response was, "We do family practice education."

When God called **Abraham**, he obeyed by faith (see Heb. 11:8-12, 17-19). The principle: *God will call you into his will for your life if you trust him enough to obey him.*

Abraham went out, not knowing where he was going. The principle: *God may send you before you can see your final destination.*

By faith Abraham traveled to a strange land, dwelling in tents. The principle: *God may place you in a strange land and outside of your comfort zone.*

Abraham looked for a city whose builder and maker was God. The principle: *God will accomplish his work by his plan and you should seek your place within it.*

Through faith Sarah (Abraham's wife) was enabled to conceive when she was past age because she believed that God would keep his promise. The principle: *God will provide whatever is necessary to accomplish his mission.*

By faith Abraham offered up Isaac because he believed that God was able to raise him up even from the dead. The principle: *God demands personal sacrifice and may even seem to demand the sacrifice of his mission as you understand it.*

The story of **Moses** also contains several biblical principles related to mission (see Ex. 3 and 4). Moses was called by God to lead the children of Israel out of Egyptian bondage and to the Promised Land. Like so many of us when challenged with a difficult or seemingly impossible task, Moses asked, "Who am I?" In other words: "Who in the world am I to do that job?"

God's answer: "I will be with you." The principle: *When God calls you, he also goes with you.*

When Moses replied that the Israelites would not listen to him, God asked, "What is in your hand?" Moses replied, "A rod" (his shepherd's tool of the trade). "Throw it on the ground," God commanded. When Moses did so, the rod turned into a serpent, which became a powerful tool and symbol of healing for all time. The principle: *Surrender "the tools of your trade" to God, and he will use them (and you) in marvelous ways.*

When I was considering the story of Moses, God spoke to my heart and said, "Do you not understand that the rod of Moses was the tool of his trade? When it was surrendered fully to me, it became my instrument to deliver a nation!"

Then I felt God ask me, "What is in your hand? Where is your rod? What are the tools of your trade?" My response was, "We do family practice education." And there it was: the incredible call to missions that God gave us! If we would fully sur-

render that to him, he would use our family medicine program (In His Image Family Practice Residency) as his rod to be a part of delivering nations.

To the best of our ability as frail human beings, we did that; and now we have fourteen graduates as long-term missionaries on the field with more in the queue to go. We have had more than six hundred participants go on more than one hundred-fifty mission trips to over forty countries. We have conducted scores of conferences and consultations.

God has been faithful to use what we surrendered to him.

–John Crouch, M.D.

As a doctor and as an individual, God has placed in your life a rod that he wants to fill with his power for his great work in redeeming the world. Have you asked God to show you that rod in your life?

VISION AND YOUR MISSION

Bruce Wilkinson, in his video series "The Vision of the Leader," describes principles related to the birth and development of a vision. A great vision begins, he says, with seeking for the need and developing, through prayer, an intentional sympathy with those in need. With cultivation, that sympathy intensifies until the passion for something to be done becomes your burden from God. God reveals to you your part in meeting that need, using your resources, skills, and talents by his grace and power. Yet you must choose to accept responsibility for that need, or not: you can answer God's call on your life, or not.

Wilkinson describes how the power for the vision comes from the closeness of our relationship with God. This requires forgiveness of our sins and obedience to Scripture. Additionally, that power becomes more effective as we claim God's promises to accomplish his mission. God may be whispering a great mission for your life, but you may be too far away to hear him, or your sin may be stuffing your ears like wet cotton. If you want a sense of mission in your life, lay your sins at the foot of the cross and leave them there; then spend time with the One who desires to call your life into significance.

And then . . . don't sit back and wait for some grand "call" to come in some supernatural form, but as Elisabeth Elliot once said, begin by realizing that God knows where he has placed us and that we are to do his work in that place. She observed that God's call to missions usually comes while Christians are already active in ministry. Each time he calls, he may show us only a part of the whole vision.

She admonished us not to wait for the big call, but to do the next thing, take the next step he has placed before us, whether big or small.

God's call to missions usually comes while Christians are already active in ministry. Each time he calls, he may show us only a part of the whole vision.

Eight guidelines for finding and fulfilling your mission:

Sometimes it may seem that some folks have been given a great and clear vision from God as if such people are special in God's plan. But God has planned and promised a mission for each of us.

1. *Realize that we all have a significant mission in kingdom work*—we need only be open to receiving it and obedient in following it. Sometimes it may seem that some folks have been given a great and clear vision from God as if such people are special in God's plan. But God has planned and promised a mission for each of us (Eph. 2:10). Christian doctors need to explore their great dreams and hopes and desires and ask God if they are not a wonderful vision from our Father to be pursued through faith (see Heb. 11:1-3).

2. *Wanting God's will is 99 percent of what is required to find God's will.* "You will seek me and find me when you seek me with all your heart" (Jer. 29:13). It is our business to seek God's will with our whole heart. It is God's business to show us clearly what that is.

3. *Our call or mission becomes most clear when we are involved in kingdom work where we are right now.* "Well done, good and faithful servant; you have been faithful over a little, I will set you over much..." (Matt. 25:21, RSV). God most often comes to us with a new, vital mission if we have proven to him through our everyday life of mission that we can be trusted.

4. *God will more likely call us to missions if we trust him to the point of obedience.* When God's call comes, the first challenge is to obey what we know to do first. God seldom reveals our whole life mission all at once. It unfolds one step at a time and our challenge is to confirm the next step as God's call and obey one step at a time. Obedience is at the heart of each step.

5. *God will likely place you in circumstances outside your comfort zone.* God likes it when we are not able to rely on our own capabilities. In missions he often keeps us off balance so we have to depend on him.

During my first trip to Albania, I was sent as an oncologist, but the chief of oncology soundly rejected my having any worthwhile purpose there. I drifted in defeat to the hematology hospital, where the chief there was arrogant and angry over the lies of previous Christian relief workers. (Note: see below for the rest of the story.)

—Al Weir, M.D.

6. *Our failures may be stepping stones to God's successes.* Only God knows what he plans to accomplish with the mission he has called us to and how this will happen. "

> For as the rain and snow come down from heaven, and return not thither but water the earth, making it bring forth and sprout, giving seed to the sower and bread to the eater, so shall my word be that goes forth from my mouth; it shall not return to me empty, but it shall accomplish that which I purpose, and prosper in the thing for which I sent it (Isa. 55:10-11, RSV).

After a week working with the chief of hematology, God transformed Dr. Xhumari's understanding of my value to him. Ten years of service and witness has followed in spite of my failure to accomplish the mission as I had planned it.
—Al Weir, M.D.

7. *God will provide the power necessary to accomplish his mission and will most visibly demonstrate his power in our weakness.* It is our business to obey; it is God's business to accomplish. "...but he said to me, 'My grace is sufficient for you, for my power is made perfect in weakness.' I will all the more gladly boast of my weaknesses, that the power of Christ may rest upon me" (2 Cor. 12:9, RSV).

Dr. Bill McCoy finished our family practice residency and remained in Tulsa practicing and teaching in our program for a couple of years. During that time, he took care of a wonderful sweet Christian lady named Jane Orr in the nursing home. When Bill felt called to the mission field, Jane Orr became a supporter in prayer and with some small amount of finances.

Dr. McCoy served a four-year term in Africa, became the medical director of the mission hospital, and then returned for furlough. He dropped by to see Jane Orr on his way to spending his furlough working and itinerating in California. Dr. McCoy owned a small house in Tulsa, the equity of which he hoped would become college money for the kids or a retirement fund, since his missionary salary was not greatly in excess of his expenses. And Bill was always generous.

But the real estate market and balloon payments had conspired to make that nest egg a cash drain rather than a revenue producer. Much of his other "savings" had gone to sustain that plan for the future.

Dr. McCoy was struggling to decide if he could really even return to the mission field, not wanting to sell the house in a down market and yet not having the cash to sustain the mortgage payments, which were in excess of the rent he was receiving.

Only God knows what he plans to accomplish with the mission he has called us to and how this will happen.

God had led him to fasting and prayer and finally he felt that God had said, "You do what I have called you to do. I will take care of the finances."

Meanwhile, after Dr. McCoy's visit, Jane Orr, now in her nineties, called me in to see her and told me God had told her to give Dr. McCoy $5,000. I said it was wonderful and asked if she could afford it, which she assured me she could. A couple of weeks later, she told me God had told her to make it $10,000. And then another few weeks later she told me God told her to make it $25,000.

Well, I talked with the nursing home administration and asked if that was feasible. Since her sister-in-law had died recently and left her some money, it was feasible, they confirmed, but suggested that she should make the gift through her will in case she needed some of the money for living or medical expenses.

Very shortly after that, she told me she had used my office to revamp her will and had left $75,000 to Dr. McCoy! I asked her if she had told him, or if I could tell him about it, and she indicated I could if I thought I should.

I called Bill and told him what had transpired. There was a stunned silence on the other end of the line and finally, in a somewhat choked voice, he recounted the struggle that he had been having about whether they would be financially able to go back to the mission field, a struggle which I didn't know about until then.

He said that about a week or so earlier, God had led him to fasting and prayer and finally he felt that God had said, "You do what I have called you to do. I will take care of the finances." And he had made the decision to return to the mission field just shortly before I called!

Bill wrote a note of thanks and blessing to Jane Orr. She called me in to see her on a Friday soon after and said she had received a note from Dr. McCoy. She asked if I would get it from her bedside stand and read it to her since she could not see very well anymore.

I did, and I had a bit of a problem reading through my tears. She was weeping with joy; and after I finished, she told me she hadn't been sure why God had left her here on this earth, that she was ready to go to be with the Lord; but maybe it was to bless Dr. McCoy.

That Sunday, two days later, Jane Orr became sick, and Monday she went home to heaven to her great reward. Mission accomplished!

God is so faithful. When people are tested in relation to their commitment to his call and prove obedient, he may just make the provision of those resources someone else's mission, to the blessing of everyone involved.

If your vision is being tested, the answer will come with faithful obedience, and God will come through in ways you have never dreamed.

—John Crouch, M.D.

8. *God's plan demands personal sacrifice.* Whether or not we are called to drop our comfortable lives and go overseas, we will not follow Christ fully without letting go of something we hold dear. German martyr Dietrich

Bonhoeffer wrote, "When Jesus calls a man, he bids him come to die." Accept your loss on the front end, and then follow the call.

Those of us who are older can look back on our lives and realize that much of our time on Earth has been spent doing good things that don't really matter in the long run. We have accumulated nice things that satisfy only temporarily and fall apart with the sands of time. We have used our skills to help people live a few years longer. We long for our lives to matter in an important and lasting way. A life that matters is exactly what God has planned for each of us and he has woven mission into the tapestry of our lives even before we were born. God has created us for mission and he is calling us to follow.

THREE QUESTIONS TO ASK YOURSELF
1. Am I living fully the mission for which God created me?
2. What dream of service has God placed on my heart?
3. What personal goals must I set aside in order to radically change my direction from "seeking temporary success" to "finding eternal significance?"

ELEVEN ACTIONS TO CONSIDER
1. Honestly seek God and ask him if you are accomplishing all that he wants you to do in your lifetime.
2. Deepen your relationship with God and ask him to share with you his heart for kingdom work that needs to be done.
3. Be involved in kingdom work/ministry right where you are now.
4. As you pray, think of the needs in your community and around the world–outside of yourself, your spouse, and your children.
5. As you identify needs that touch your heart and as you dream of what could be, answer the question, "What 'rod' (tool of my trade) has God placed in my hand?"
6. As God lays it on your heart to do something, be quick to obey and take the next step – whether it is only a small one, or even if it is such a great one that it will disrupt your life.
7. Trust God to confirm his call to the degree you need it.
8. Remember the steps of Abraham's faith as he pursued God's call.
9. Always be prepared to give "your" ministry to God. Do his work, and don't possess it.
10. Trust God to care for those you love as you follow his call.
11. Explore CMDA missions opportunities.

Dietrich Bonhoeffer wrote, "When Jesus calls a man, he bids him come to die." Accept your loss on the front end, and then follow the call.

PRAYER

Father,
I thank you for saving us and calling us to be a part of your plan to bring your
kingdom to the earth. I thank you that each of us has a mission to accomplish that
will advance your kingdom, bring us fulfillment, and bless our families. I pray
that your Spirit will speak to our hearts with a clear call. Give us your grace and
courage to be quickly obedient. I pray for clear direction each step of the way. I
pray that you will shape and mold our character and provide all the skills we need
to gain resources and recruit partners to accomplish the mission. Give us a fresh,
new, exciting vision that will impact the world. All this we pray in Jesus' name.

–Amen

Ethics

*J*erry *was an engineering student who planned to go to the mission field. While in university, he spent his free time volunteering as leader of the junior high youth group at church. After a fun couple of hours riding ATVs on trails through the woods, he led the kids on a shortcut back to the parking lot as dusk was approaching. He didn't see the guy-wire as he circled around the power pole, and it hit him in the neck, knocking him off his vehicle. One of the youngsters used her cell phone to call 911. The paramedics found him pulseless and not breathing. Vigorous resuscitation on the scene and in the ED restored his circulation. But he never regained awareness.*

His parents and sister spent untold hours at his bedside, and their prayers for his recovery were supplemented by extended family and friends. After he stabilized, he was admitted to a rehabilitation unit for several weeks. However, after three months, his physician, also a believer, declared that Jerry was in a permanent vegetative state with an almost zero chance of any improvement. His family took him home for long-term care.

Jerry's mother was a nurse. She stopped working to care for him. His married sister lived nearby and helped. His father also learned the routines. For the next seven years Jerry's family hoped and prayed for the unexpected—"just some sign that he knows we're here, Lord." Slowly, they accepted that he would never improve, and his mother and sister began to talk with the doctor about whether it would ever be okay to stop his life support since they knew he would not want to continue to exist in this condition. The only life support he was on was a feeding tube. His father was reluctant to stop his feedings, asking, "What will we tell the neighbors he died from?"

How should this faithful family decide whether they should continue to provide artificially administered fluids and nutrition for Jerry, or whether

Do Christians use the same methods as non-Christians? Do all Christians use the same method? Is there a biblical approach that gives "the right answer"?

they should stop this form of life support with the expectation that he would die?

METHODS OF MORAL REASONING

Many medical decisions are practical clinical decisions based on an assessment of data such as which test or which treatment is most likely to give the best result in this case? In these situations, the healthcare professional's responsibility is to report the best available information on benefits, risks, and burdens of the proposal, and often to make a recommendation. It is then the responsibility of the patient (or surrogate decision maker) to make a decision based on the patient's values and wishes. This is a joint effort of professional and patient.

Some medical decisions are also moral decisions, including such considerations as: What is the right thing to do? What are the values involved, and which takes priority? How do healthcare professionals, patients, and families make moral decisions in medicine? How do they decide what is right or wrong, good or bad? What if the professional and the patient or surrogate have different moral values or use different methods of reasoning? Do Christians use the same methods as non-Christians? Do all Christians use the same method? Is there a biblical approach that gives "the right answer"?

The four most common methods of moral reasoning are principles, virtue, consequences, and casuistry.

Principle-Based Moral Reasoning

The most popular method of teaching medical ethics is principalism, which looks for rules to help guide moral decisions.

Secular medical ethics teaches four primary principles of decision making in medicine:

- ◆Non-maleficence - first of all, do no harm;
- ◆Beneficence - do what is good for the patient;
- ◆Autonomy - patients have a right to self-determination;
- ◆Justice - treat like patients alike.

These fundamental principles can be very helpful as professionals and patients struggle to do the right thing. However, focusing on different principles can lead to different conclusions.

For example, in situations like Jerry's (a) some would interpret the principle of non-maleficence to suggest that we should not remove the feeding tube because it will knowingly lead to a patient's death, which is always bad; (b) others might focus on beneficence, believing that removing the feeding tube would be good since it would release him from the permanent vegetative state, which they believe is worse than death; (c) others would focus on autonomy and would try to learn what Jerry would want if he knew he was in this situation; (d) others would argue, based on justice, that we should develop a policy so that all patients in a permanent vegetative state are treated the same, taking into consideration the amount of resources being used.

This principle-based method of reasoning may be less than totally helpful when two principles are in conflict and you are unable to follow both. A trivial example: Should you immunize your children? Beneficence says you should protect your children from terrible diseases when possible. But non-maleficence says you should do no harm, and you do cause harm by immunizing (pain of injection; frequent minor side effects; rare serious complications). Autonomy would allow the child to refuse the immunization. Justice would suggest that all (or at least most) children should be immunized to create herd immunity. Though the answer to this question seems obvious, principles alone cannot dictate that answer.

In our secular society, the principle of autonomy has gained prominence, even predominance. Autonomy trumps all other considerations in the minds of many. Is that consistent with biblical teaching? Christians generally accept these four principles, but may have a different way to apply them when two or more are in conflict. In addition, believers can use other biblical principles as they struggle with such decisions, including the following:

◆God's sovereignty - God has ultimate authority over life and death (Rom. 9:19-24); both in life and in death we are his (Rom. 14:8).
◆Obedience - In both the Old Testament (Deut. 6:18; 7:12) and the New Testament (John 13:17; 15:10) we are taught that God's blessing is contingent on our obedience.
◆Free will - We are free to accept and follow God's teachings or not. However, Christians do not accept the popular secular notion that personal autonomy is almost absolute since Scripture teaches that there are some constraints on human choices.
◆Dominion - In his exquisite creation, God gave dominion to humankind (Gen. 1:26). This suggests that we have at least some authority to shape life as caretakers of his property, including, by implication, our bodies.
◆Stewardship - Along with dominion come responsibility and accountability. We should live healthy lifestyles, seek medical care when needed, and

This principle-based method of reasoning may be less than totally helpful when two principles are in conflict and you are unable to follow both.

*Principles
are important
from both a
secular and
Christian
perspective.
But sometimes
they do not
give a clearly
right or
wrong
answer.*

use our natural and synthetic resources wisely. We are not our own, we are bought with a price (1 Cor. 6:19-20). Our body is the temple of the Holy Spirit (1 Cor. 3:16), and we are called to offer our bodies as a living sacrifice (Rom. 12:1).

♦Sanctity of human life - The sacredness of human life is a biblical principle that is not articulated in a single verse, but is clearly demonstrated throughout Scripture. It includes the critical concept of the *imago Dei*, the image of God present in each person (Gen. 1:27).

♦Eternal life - This earthly life is not the end, but is merely a prelude to an eternal life of worshipping and praising God.

♦Meritorious suffering - Sometimes God expects us to choose to suffer rather than to take the easy road (Heb. 11:24-25), anticipating a glorious future (Rom. 8:18-21). Paul finally accepted his "thorn in the flesh," as he understood that "God's grace is sufficient" (2 Cor. 12:8-9).

♦Contentment - We are encouraged to be content in whatever situation we find ourselves (Phil. 4:11). At the same time, we may use our own efforts and prayer for God's help as we try to improve our situation.

♦Others - There are other principles of daily living found in Scripture, which may have bearing on specific situations and specific decisions.

The primary difference between the secular and Christian perspectives is that the former is person-centered, and the latter should be God-centered. John Kilner has pointed out that, in addition to being God-centered, the believer's approach to difficult decisions about life and death must be "reality bounded" and "love impelled."[1]

How would these additional scriptural principles help Jerry's family and physician with the decision about continued use of his feeding tube? Yes, God is sovereign, but outcomes are often dependent on human decisions. So how do we differentiate between what is God's will and what is our own selfish desire? We have dominion over much of nature, and we are to be stewards of our lives and our resources. In showing respect for the sanctity of human life, the imago Dei *in each person, how far do we go in preventing death?*

When it is clear that Jerry will never again have awareness, are we preventing him from receiving his eternal reward by postponing his death? On the other hand, should we continue to provide loving care for him in spite of his lack of awareness in order to demonstrate to others the preciousness of human life regardless of its quality?

Principles are important from both a secular and Christian perspective. But sometimes they do not give a clearly right or wrong answer. And different individuals, relying on human reasoning, scriptural application, or prayerful direction, may arrive at different conclusions. Does this mean one is right and one is wrong? Are there other methods that may help?

Virtue

While principles are about doing the right thing, virtue is about being the right kind of person. Professional virtue has been an important part of the practice of medicine for centuries. And from a Christian perspective, the presence of the Holy Spirit in the life of a believer is expected to make that person more virtuous, more Christlike. So "virtue ethics" also deserves a prominent place in both secular and Christian reasoning.

Edmund Pellegrino, M.D., is the most prominent proponent of virtue as the key to making moral decisions in medicine. He and co-author David Thomasma have written a series of books on the topic; two are pertinent to our discussion here, one about the place of virtue in medicine and the other focused specifically on the Christian virtues.

In *The Virtues in Medical Practice*[2] Pellegrino and Thomasma devote a chapter to each of the following virtues they believe to be foundational to the practice of medicine:

*Fidelity to Trust
*Compassion
*Phronesis (practical wisdom)
*Justice
*Fortitude
*Temperance
*Integrity
*Self-effacement.

In *The Christian Virtues in Medical Practice*,[3] they add content on the matters of faith, hope, and charity, integrating these with the foundational principles of medical ethics.

Jerry's family has demonstrated fidelity, compassion, fortitude, integrity, and self-effacement for more than seven years. When, if ever, should questions of practical wisdom enter the picture?

As it becomes increasingly clear that he will never awaken, do issues of stewardship and personal values allow changing goals from survival to no longer postponing death by mechanical interventions?

While principles are about doing the right thing, virtue is about being the right kind of person.

Consequences

In addition to principles and virtues, many consider, or even rely upon, anticipated consequences in making moral decisions. It is not only natural to look at the consequences of our actions for guidance in making decisions, it is imperative to do so. That is part of the warp and woof of medicine. Professionals and patients should not suggest or agree to a particular course of action without serious consideration of the consequences. Consequential reasoning dominates secular medicine. This is so important that we sometimes think only of consequences, overlooking the requirements of principles and virtue.

It is consideration of the consequences of an unwanted or untimely pregnancy that has led to societal and professional acceptance of abortion. A young woman unexpectedly becomes pregnant and fears this will interfere with her career plans. Looking primarily at the consequences, it is attractive for her to accept the dominant principle of autonomy. She may accept the principle of the sanctity of human life. She may understand that the developing fetus is a person. She may realize that termination of her pregnancy will cause irreversible harm to that fetal person. But the self-centered approach that is so much a part of human nature may lead her, often with the recommendation of others, to accept the "better consequences" of ending the pregnancy.

This consequential approach to medical decisions, based on the predominance of autonomy, is relatively new in society and in medicine.

This consequential approach to medical decisions, based on the predominance of autonomy, is relatively new in society and in medicine. The forsaking (or at least ignoring) of principles and virtues in order to focus on consequences, then making decisions based on what consequences the individual prefers, has very quickly become very popular in society as a whole and in medicine.

Christians will recognize that an expression of absolute autonomy is the central element of the sinful nature of human beings (Gen. 3:1-4). Many who recognize this are so focused on the evil human nature that they are unwilling to even consider consequences as a guide in their decision making. Such an individual might focus primarily on the sanctity of human life and refuse to weigh the consequences of following this principle. But we cannot ignore consequences. In fact, Jesus admonishes us to carefully count the cost while making plans so we will not be ridiculed if our plans don't work out (Luke 14:28-29).

In contemplating the decision about Jerry's feeding tube, a focus only on the principle of the sanctity of life might lead some believers to be unwilling to remove the tube. That same narrow focus could also lead some to insist on using dialysis if he should develop kidney failure or even a ventilator if he was unable to breathe adequately on his own. This vitalistic approach – i.e., focusing on only the principle of the sanctity of human life, and insisting on preserving biological life regardless of the quality of that life or the consequences of preserving it – overlooks several balancing tenets of the faith.

We must recognize this Christian bias against consequentialistic reasoning based on our understanding of human nature. Theologian John Feinberg has suggested, however, that there are several situations when Christians are allowed or even required to consider consequences when using the more traditional principle-based and virtue-based reasoning:

♦when there are no moral absolutes for or against an action, the decision must be prudential, i.e., it must consider the consequences;
♦when there is a conflict of duties and both may not be fulfilled, an assessment of probable consequences may make one choice morally preferable to another;
♦when there are limited resources, an assessment of consequences may help determine that one choice is preferable to another.[4]

Thomas Aquinas recognized that sometimes a good act can produce an unintended bad consequence; his "rule of double effect" allows such an action if several criteria are met, and this clearly requires an assessment of the probable consequences.[5]

When we know our moral duty (e.g., the Golden Rule), but are not sure how to apply it in a given situation, an assessment of the anticipated consequences may give guidance.

Christian principles and virtues give important guidance in moral decision making, but do not always give clarity about "the right answer." In those cases, weighing consequences may be necessary, and may sometimes be sufficient to resolve the dilemma.

Casuistry

Casuistry is "the method of analyzing and resolving instances of moral perplexity by interpreting general moral rules in light of particular circumstances."[6] This name was coined in the seventeenth century as a pejorative term to describe those who discussed "cases of conscience." The implication was often that casuists were loose with Scripture, principles, and virtues. For several centuries, casuistry had a poor reputation, often being mistaken for "relativism" or "situation ethics."

We must recognize this Christian bias against consequentialistic reasoning based on our understanding of human nature. Christian principles and virtues give important guidance in moral decision making, but do not always give clarity about "the right answer."

We do not always "follow the rules," often because they do not give a clear answer in a particular case.

However, the concept has achieved a more respectable position as a valid method of moral reasoning since an in-depth study and defense by philosophers Jonsen and Toulmin.[7] One of the reasons this method has become popular in contemporary philosophy and in medical ethics is because it is the way that most of us think most of the time, especially when making difficult treatment decisions in complicated cases. We do not always "follow the rules," often because they do not give a clear answer in a particular case.

One of the characteristics of casuistic reasoning is that it uses paradigm cases to help sort out what is best in a current case. For example, suppose we are trying to decide whether to do a heart transplant for a thirty-five-year-old woman who is dying from an incurable viral infection of her heart muscle.

Let's consider two paradigm cases where the decision seems clear: (a) an infant with an irreparable lethal heart condition who is otherwise healthy; there is a donor heart available; her parents are willing to take on the complicated post-op care; and, they have adequate insurance coverage (b) an eighty-five-year-old man with advanced dementia and widespread cancer is also in irreversible heart failure; he has no one to care for him post-op; and, he has inadequate insurance coverage.

Should we do transplants in these cases? Clearly it would be the right thing to do in case (a), but it would not be justified in case (b). So we then ask, how does our thirty-five-year-old woman compare to these two paradigms?

What makes her case similar to or different from each? Such considerations might make it easier to decide for her.

The important thing to remember about casuistry is that it does not ignore the rules or the virtues or the consequences. It uses all three, but it may apply them differently, or give them a different prioritization, in different cases. The danger of casuistic reasoning is that it offers nothing beyond the case by which to judge the case.

APPLICATIONS OF THESE METHODS OF MORAL REASONING[8]

Decisions based on Principles

Case A: Mary is a twenty-one-year-old college senior. Based on her excellent academic performance, she has been offered a full scholarship for graduate training in her chosen field of American history. She unexpectedly and unhappily finds she is eight weeks pregnant just at the time she must accept or decline the scholarship, which cannot be deferred.

♦Many non-Christians and some Christians believe that Mary's autonomy is predominant, and she is free to choose whether to continue the pregnancy or accept the scholarship.

♦Most Christians and some non-Christians believe that the sanctity of human life, even fetal life, forbids terminating the pregnancy. Some would further believe she is obligated to raise the child, while others would accept that her choice to continue the pregnancy would not preclude the option of adoption and attendance at graduate school with alternative funding at a later date.

Case B: Roland is an eighty-three-year-old retired farmer with long-standing lung disease. He has been in respiratory failure twice in the past year. Both times, treatment for a few days on a ventilator in the ICU allowed him to get enough better to go home, though he is now bed-bound, dependent on oxygen, and chronically short of breath. He is in the ED again with a severe pneumonia and unable to breathe adequately. He says he doesn't want to go back to the ICU or to be put on the ventilator. He is ready to accept that he is dying and only requests sufficient medication to keep him comfortable.

♦Most Christians and non-Christians would agree that, as long as Roland clearly understands the options and the consequences, it is ethically permissible for him to exercise his autonomy to decline potentially death-postponing treatment if he feels the burdens of treatment and of continued life outweigh the benefits.

Decisions based on Virtue

Case C: Rebecca is a forty-six-year-old single mother of two teenagers. She has been battling an aggressive cancer of her pancreas for several months, accepting major surgery, radiation, and chemotherapy. The cancer is now widespread and is exceedingly painful. Her physician has been making frequent house calls, rapidly increasing her doses of narcotics to try to make her remaining days tolerable. She is still in awful pain and is unable to sleep.

Today she asks her trusted physician for a large prescription of sleeping pills. They talk about her desire to die soon and her plan to take an overdose to end her life quickly.

Today she asks her physician for a large prescription of sleeping pills. They talk about her desire to die soon and her plan to take an overdose to end her life quickly.

◆Most Christians and many non-Christians believe that professional virtue of fidelity to trust requires a physician faced with this request to (a) redouble efforts at pain control, including requesting consultation from a pain specialist, and (b) decline to change roles from healer to assistant in suicide. If all efforts fail to control the pain, most agree that it would be ethically permissible to give the patient sufficient medication to render her unconscious (palliative sedation), even if this means that she might die more quickly from dehydration.

◆Some non-Christians and a few Christians believe that the obligation to the virtue of compassion would allow a physician to honor Rebecca's request to intentionally hasten her death.

Decisions based on Consequences

Case D: Dr. Bradley is a cardiothoracic surgeon who is active in an adult heart transplant program. He currently has two patients on the waiting list. Ralph is sixty-one and has had three heart attacks so that his heart muscle is irreparably damaged; he is at home where his congestive heart failure confines him to bed; he will probably not live for more than a few weeks or months unless he gets a heart transplant. Beverly is twenty-four and has been in the ICU on major life-support for three weeks because a viral infection has irreversibly damaged her heart muscle; she will probably die in a few days without a heart transplant. Dr. Bradley is notified that a donor heart has become available and there is a good tissue match for either Ralph or Beverly. Which patient should get the heart?

◆Dr. Bradley has an equal obligation to seek the best treatment for both of these patients. However, most people would agree that in this case of limited resources, Beverly should get this heart primarily because she is in more imminent danger of death, but also because she has a longer projected survival time if the transplant is successful. While using age as a determining factor is rarely justified because it is discriminatory, it may be justified when we are dealing with an absolutely scarce resource.

Decisions made through Casuistry

In truth, there was likely some casuistic thinking involved in each of the above cases, even though principles, virtues, or consequences seemed to dominate in different cases.

The case of Jerry that opened this chapter is a good place to apply casuistry. Should his family continue to provide loving nursing care, fluids, and nutrition, or may they withdraw artificially administered sustenance with the expectation that he will die in several days?

♦Most people find this a tough decision without a clearly right or wrong answer. Most non-Christians would say it is ethically permissible to withdraw the feeding tube based on (a) autonomy - his previously stated wish to not be maintained in a state of unawareness, (b) non-maleficence - it is wrong to keep him alive in this condition "worse than death," (c) justice - the cost of continued care for this patient with no discernable quality of life, or (d) the virtues of compassion, practical wisdom, and self-effacement.

♦Many Christians would agree that it is acceptable to stop the feeding tube, relying on these principles and virtues, and adding the concepts of stewardship, dominion, and a belief in God's sovereignty and eternal life.

♦Other Christians would offer the biblical principle of the sanctity of human life as a reason that his life must be extended since this can be accomplished with minimal effort or cost, he is not "terminally ill," and life with no perceptible quality is still inherently worthwhile. Some Christians would support Jerry's dad for being reluctant to withdraw his feeding tube, but would criticize his consequential reasoning as being weak or self-centered ("What will the neighbors think?").

It is tempting to think that if believers search Scripture thoroughly and deny personal biases, we could all come to the same conclusion about "the right thing to do" in all cases. This should happen in some cases where treatment options are clearly within God's will or not, but it is not going to happen in all cases.

Based on our discussion, it is even safe to say that two Christians may earnestly seek God's will in a given case and come to different conclusions, each believing he or she has "the answer."

But searching for the answer must allow room for differing interpretation of principles, virtues, and circumstances when the decision maker is guided by a passionate search for the will of God through prayer and Christian counsel.

Many Christians would agree that it is acceptable to stop the feeding tube, relying on these principles and virtues, and adding the concepts of stewardship, dominion, and a belief in God's sovereignty and eternal life.

PRACTICAL SUGGESTIONS

Some physicians are reluctant to make recommendations, believing their responsibility is merely to lay out the options, letting the patient's autonomy lead to a personal choice as in a cafeteria. However, part of the responsibility of the professional is to give guidance, based on the patient's values and wishes.

♦Get the facts - Good medicine begins with good facts. Good ethics begins with good facts. Good moral reasoning also begins with good facts. We can't hope to come to the best possible decision if our starting point is less clear than is humanly possible.

♦Clarify the options and likely outcomes - Since prognosis is not factual, it is often wise to get two or more opinions about likely outcomes.

♦Identify the appropriate decision maker - If the patient is unable or unwilling to make the treatment decision, determine who the appropriate surrogate is. Still involve others in the discussion and try to reach consensus, but look to the surrogate for a decision if there is no consensus.

♦Elicit values - Learn the temporal and eternal values of the patient and family. Involve the patient's pastor, priest, or rabbi, or a hospital chaplain.

♦Make recommendations - Some physicians are reluctant to do this, believing their responsibility is merely to lay out the options, letting the patient's autonomy lead to a personal choice as in a cafeteria. However, part of the responsibility of the professional is to give guidance, based on the patient's values and wishes. In some situations, two or more options may be equally valid from both a clinical and moral standpoint, but in others, clinical judgment clearly suggests one over another. Of course the patient or surrogate is free to ignore a physician's recommendation, but this does not negate the physician's responsibility to make one.

♦Seek consultation - In difficult cases, second clinical opinions, consultation with an ethics committee or clinical ethicist, and counsel from clergy may all help to clarify the best thing to do.

♦Pray - Individual prayer is always appropriate for the believing physician. Offering to pray with a patient or family is almost always appropriate when caring for people of similar faith, and sometimes even with patients who deny a spiritual faith. It is also helpful to involve the patient's faith community in prayer, not only for healing, but also for guidance.

♦Recognize the method of moral reasoning you are using - It is often helpful to articulate the principles, virtues, or consequences on which you are relying.

•Allow time - Difficult treatment decisions can rarely be made quickly. Allow time for the patient or family to hear and process the information; allow time for the patient's body to clarify the prognosis; allow time for different individuals to work through the issues, realizing that different people will likely come to conclusions at different times; allow time to pray; allow time for the Holy Spirit to bring peace, comfort, and resolution.

THREE QUESTIONS TO ASK YOURSELF
1. Which method of moral reasoning do I find myself using most often?
2. What would I do about the feeding tube if I were Jerry's family? His physician?
3. What should I do as a physician if my patient's right to autonomy conflicts with my principle of sanctity of life?

THREE ACTIONS TO CONSIDER
1. Memorize the four methods of moral reasoning.
2. Search this week for a case in your practice or that of your colleagues where you can apply these methods in ethical decision making.
3. Consider with prayer whether you should start or join an ethics committee in your hospital.

PRAYER

Our Father,

We thank you for who you are, for how you love us, and for how you continue to be involved in our lives. We bring before you now the situation of [this patient] for your guidance. We thank you for his [her] life. We thank you for the capabilities of modern medicine. But we confess our limitations, both of our technical abilities, and of our human reasoning.

We ask you now for two things: We pray first for your wisdom, that the Holy Spirit would clarify our understanding, our thoughts, and our ideas, and that your will be done. Second, we pray for the peace that passes all understanding. You are the not the author of confusion, but of peace. We ask that as your will becomes clear, we would have your peace that we can accept the direction that you impress upon our hearts and the outcome that is your will.

We pray this in the name above all names, the name of Jesus.

—Amen

NOTES:

1. John F. Kilner. *Life on the Line*. Grand Rapids, Mich.: Eerdmans, 1992; 349 pp.

2. Edmund D. Pellegrino and David C. Thomasma. New York: Oxford University Press, 1993; 205 pp.

3. Edmund D. Pellegrino and David C. Thomasma. Washington, D.C.: Georgetown University Press, 1996; 164 pp.

4. Adapted from a lecture at "The Christian Stake in Bioethics" conference, Deerfield, Ill., May 20, 1994.

5. Aquinas' criteria: (a) the initial act must be inherently good or at least morally neutral; (b) the bad consequence may be foreseen, but not intended; (c) the good effect may not be achieved by means of the bad consequence; (d) there must be a proportionately grave reason for allowing the bad consequence; (e) there must be no other way to achieve the good effect.

6. *Encyclopedia of Bioethics*, Revised edition, Vol 1. WT Reich, editor; New York: Macmillan, 1995:344.

7. *The Abuse of Casuistry: A History of Moral Reasoning*. Albert R. Jonsen and Stephen Toulmin. Berlkey: University of California Press, 1988.

8. Editorial note: the following are examples that demonstrate the application of these methods in given ethical situations. The conclusions reached in these examples do not imply our endorsement of those conclusions.

Managing Time

*D*oug had been in practice two years, and generally enjoyed his work, but he struggled with one thing: time. Medicine was his calling. He was attracted to the sciences in high school, and by the time he entered college, he knew what he wanted to do. He enjoyed the pre-med curriculum. Excellent grades came naturally to him, such that he had a choice of medical schools. He worked hard in med school and residency because he loved what he was doing. When it was time to enter practice, he was ready.

Joining a group, Doug quickly encountered some of the things med school didn't teach him like coding and billing processes, managing employees, and having to think about business and financial issues with the practice. He focused on practicing medicine as he had been trained, and tried to leave those other issues to the more seasoned members of his group. His wake-up call came at the end of the second year.

Doug's partners had been patient with him as he oriented himself to private practice. He had a salary guarantee from the hospital in the first year, so they didn't pay much attention to his productivity. They graciously and patiently encouraged him to pick up the pace as he plodded along, not wanting to upset him since he was providing excellent medical care to his patients and lightening their burden for taking call.

But by the end of the second year, when it was time for him to be offered an ownership position in the practice, the group could no longer ignore the obvious. Doug was a poor manager of his time. He wasn't carrying his own weight. In spite of his excellent medical skills, he was struggling to stay in business. His love of medicine was not enough to sustain a viable practice.

If he wanted his place as a partner in the practice, it was time for him to learn new skills; it was time to learn time management.

We can't expand the clock; we can only manage our efforts within the boundaries of time.

Doug is not alone. Time is a natural limit everyone has to deal with. We can't expand the clock; we can only manage our efforts within the boundaries of time. Some people are more adept at it than others. Personal productivity in every field ranges widely, and the variance in medicine and dentistry is no exception. Data from national surveys demonstrate that doctors at the seventy-fifth percentile of production often see twice as many patients as those at the twenty-fifth percentile, even though they both work roughly the same number of weeks per year.

What is the difference in the practice of these two groups of doctors? Are the less productive doctors better listeners and more careful providers, or are they just less efficient in their use of time? We all need more time, whether or not God asks us to fill that time with more patient care.

The motives for learning time management skills go beyond the desire to increase personal income. Christian practitioners have more reasons than most to manage their time wisely. Higher productivity may provide opportunity for greater generosity to missions. It also allows practitioners to take more time for mission trips, to mentor Christian medical students, to serve the poor in the local community, and to do a better job of caring for their patients within a practice limited by time constraints. Many Christians view time management as a stewardship issue, like money, and seek to honor the Lord in the way they structure their activities – and feel guilty when they don't. Richard Swenson, M.D., makes the strongest case for time management in his book, *Margin*, on the grounds of physical, spiritual, and emotional health.[1]

FOUNDATION

For some reason, God has placed us within the boundaries of time on this side of heaven. God does not make a mess of things, so, if we are overwhelmed, the problem is our doing. He has created us for a life of joy, ministry and family, so if we have lost these blessings due to time pressures, it is likely that he would like to help us find them again. It is also likely that fixing our time problem is not possible without God's help and that he is more likely to help us if we are working towards his will for time in our lives.

What then is God's will for the use of our time? The apostle Paul sums it up best in Eph. 1:9-10: "And he made known to us the mystery of his will according to his good pleasure, which he purposed in Christ, to be put into effect when the times will have reached their fulfillment – to bring all things in heaven and on earth together under one head, even Christ."

When time is finally fulfilled, the world will be one with Christ as our King. Therefore, as we seek to reorder our time, and seek God's help in doing so, keep in mind that the redemption of the world provides the context upon which we make all of our decisions. We must look at the time available to us as an instrument handed to us by God to redeem his world. We must then mold our use of it according to that purpose.

The fact that God gives us time for his purpose means that there is plenty of it to accomplish his goals for our lives. We need not worry how short our days or how few our years may be. God is able and willing to complete all of the work he has allotted for us within the time he has allotted to us, as Paul wrote: "being confident of this, that he who began a good work in you will carry it on to completion until the day of Christ Jesus" (Phil. 1:6).

Using time responsibly is our business. Getting the work done successfully is God's, and he's got the power to do it. The proper foundation for the use of my time is God's purpose with God's power. So, how do I go about fixing the chaotic hectic schedule of my life according to God's plan?

Managing time wisely is vital to achieving our goals, to attaining the time, money, and accomplishments necessary to fulfill God's purpose for our lives. The habits of good time management can be our servants, enabling us to work toward personal and professional goals more efficiently and effectively. They become a means to an end. The reward for applying the discipline of time management is the freedom to choose how we will spend our time. We may choose in God's will to devote more time to individual patient care, service to others, devotion to God, self-care and family relationships, or to any other activity that feeds our soul and pleases him.

Managing time wisely is not a problem to solve. It is a polarity to manage.[2] It requires persistent attention to competing demands and regular discernment of the priorities of those demands for your time and attention. Managing time wisely in one circumstance does not solve how you will manage your time when that circumstance recurs. Each situation requires a new decision, but the discipline becomes more natural with experience and with knowledge of the basic tools used by those who are most effective in managing their time.

"Sometimes you have to stop running long enough to build a bicycle," as the saying goes. That's the promise of time management training. It takes a little effort to learn, but it helps you get where you want to go faster, and gives you the option of going further in the same amount of time you had in which to run.

The Pareto Principle

Managing time wisely takes more than the right motivation. It requires skills that can be learned by understanding the underlying principles, mastering the basic tools, and consistently applying the discipline required to

The fact that God gives us time for his purpose means that there is plenty of it to accomplish his goals for our lives.

The Pareto Principle would indicate that we spend about 20 percent of our time accomplishing 80 percent of our results.

be successful. The goal of wise time management is to gain efficiencies that enable you to accomplish more than would be possible without paying attention to time. Greater efficiency gets converted to greater effectiveness. You work smarter, not harder. You achieve more in less time. That frees up time to be reapplied at your discretion. It does not expand the clock. It expands your personal effectiveness.

In 1906, Italian economist Vilfredo Pareto described his observation about the distribution of wealth in a mathematical formula. He argued that in all countries and all times, about 20 percent of the people own about 80 percent of the wealth. Over the years, Pareto's Law has proved remarkably resilient in empirical studies. After Pareto made his observation, many others began to observe similar relationships in other disciplines. The Pareto Principle stuck, and is now widely recognized for its management wisdom.

Applied to time, the Pareto Principle would indicate that we spend about 20 percent of our time accomplishing 80 percent of our results. The flip side, of course, is that we use 80 percent rather inefficiently to accomplish only 20 percent of our achievements. Therefore, if we could understand what we do differently in the 20 percent of our time that we are highly efficient, and applied those thought and activity patterns to a greater portion of our schedule, we could accomplish greater results in the same amount of time. If we get a four-fold return on our effectiveness 20 percent of the time, then being efficient 30 percent of the time could have the impact of enabling us to accomplish 140 percent of what we formerly expected of ourselves. Of course, all of this is theoretical and nearly impossible to measure with accuracy for any given individual, but the hope of greater efficiency and effectiveness is appealing nonetheless. The clear benefit of the so-called Pareto Principle is that it focuses our attention on the portion of our time when we are most productive, challenges us to learn the lessons we take for granted in those periods, and to apply them to other periods of our schedule.

TIME MANAGEMENT TOOLS

The tools of time management are simple and almost free. They can be constructed with paper and pencil. Three tools that can aid in managing time wisely are an activity log, a to-do list, and a system of prioritizing activities. Once the tools are understood, there are tactics for refining their use and for applying the principles of time management in specific circumstances. As we explore these tools and tactics, the assumption is that they will be applied to work routines, but they can be equally valuable in evaluating time usage outside of work.

Activity Log

The first step in managing time wisely is to evaluate your habits and activity patterns by tracking them for a typical week. You can construct a simple activity log, which builds on the Pareto Principle and gives you the opportunity to examine how you currently spend your time. You should track your time in fifteen-minute intervals to gain the most complete picture of your habits and routines. Prepare a page for each day and make a note of your activities as they happen. If you try to remember how you spent your day retrospectively, you will likely forget details or be inaccurate in recording them.

If the bulk of your time is spent in office visits, you may want to note the number of patients seen in your office visit time as well as what you did for them or the type of services provided. Keep it simple, describing the activity in the briefest of forms. Entering information in the log should not be a time-consuming burden in itself. Less than a minute per entry should be plenty.

After you have documented a week's activities, take time to analyze it. You may want to categorize your time into segments like these:

*direct patient care in the office
*direct patient care in the hospital
*traveling between service locations
*documentation time
*communicating with others – staff, colleagues, pharmacies, hospital staff
*administrative time
*personal development – continuing education, reading

Examine what percentage of time you spent in each category. Notice what surprises you about your work patterns as well as what is particularly satisfying. Pay attention to the time of day and the types of activities in which you felt most effective. Write down your analytical observations so you can reflect on them, and begin to form plans about changing your work habits toward more efficient and effective outcomes. No one else needs to see your activity log or your analysis. This introspective exercise is for your personal benefit only. It is designed to inform you, to help you become aware of your thought patterns and habits so you can increase your stewardship of time.

You may also want to compare your time analysis with your expectations for yourself. Most professionals, especially self-employed professionals like physicians and dentists, don't have written job descriptions, but we all

The first step in managing time wisely is to evaluate your habits and activity patterns by tracking them for a typical week.

have a sense about what activities help us achieve our goals. Compare the time-usage patterns you observe to your goals. Is your time aligned with your intentions? Are there activities that can be eliminated or minimized through delegation to free you up for more of the activities that are vital to your goals? As you begin to critique your current use of time, you'll most likely identify specific activities that are more satisfying and more important than others in helping you attain your personal and professional goals.

To-Do List

Once you have oriented yourself to your current work patterns and to the activities that are most vital to your success – however you define it – you will be ready to deploy the next tool, the to-do list. A to-do list may seem irrelevant when your work patterns are predictable and consistent from day to day, but those who manage multiple roles and a wide variety of tasks find lists invaluable. To use it fully, update it daily. You may want to devote the first ten minutes of each day to maintaining your to-do list. You may be surprised at the breadth of tasks you actually encounter in a typical day.

A to-do list can be constructed from the same material as the activity log–paper and pencil. A list can also be developed and maintained on a computer or personal digital assistant (PDA), using Microsoft Outlook™ or an equivalent software product. Plain paper offers more format flexibility, but those who rely on technology for other functions may prefer to integrate their to-do list with their other work tools.

Prepare four columns with the following headings:

Priority	Activity	Deadline	Time Required

Identify activities that can be completed in the amount of time you consider as a traditional (comfortable) workday of maybe eight to ten hours. List those activities you intend to accomplish in the second column as you think of them. Don't worry about the order. That analysis will come later. The first step is to simply capture every activity you can think of that you intend to perform in the next few days or weeks to help you attain your overall goals. Some activities will reflect short-term goals while others may reflect long-term intentions. You may want to break down large long-term goals into smaller pieces. For example, if you have a goal of making a clinical presentation, list separate activities for constructing the outline, researching specific components, preparing the slides, and making the actual presentation. A few activities may seem implausible but interesting.

Write them down anyway. Let the construction of your to-do list be like brainstorming, devoid of critical judgments, at least initially.

Use the deadline column to identify the date each activity needs to be accomplished by, based on the expectations of others. If there are no deadlines imposed on you by others for certain activities, create a self-imposed deadline that reflects your ambitions.

In the last column, note your estimate of the time required to accomplish each item on your list. Some activities may be accomplished in minutes like phone calls or making appointments. Others may require hours, such as meetings or drafting an extensive written document. Give it your best estimate, understanding that your accuracy may be way off initially. Logging your expectations will be important to managing your time the way you intend to, the way that is aligned with your goals. Later you can use these projections to evaluate your time management skills.

When you think about your life, what within it is really important for you to accomplish?

Prioritization

When you think about your life, what within it is really important for you to accomplish? When one doctor sat down and looked at his own life the following list emerged:

1. Worship
2. Family
3. Friends
4. Witness
5. Medical Work
6. Service to the Poor and Suffering
7. Study
8. Recreation
9. Personal Accomplishments
10. Teaching and Mentoring
11. Health Maintenance
12. Church Fellowship

These are the things that doctor needed to be doing in order to live the way that makes sense to him within God's plan. Each of these categories should then lead to certain activities in his or her life that all flow from the foundational purpose of working as God's servant to redeem the world. Some of the categories on the surface may seem secular, while others seem spiritual; but, if we understand our foundational purpose correctly, every category should be filled with the presence and purpose of God. None is

Deciding how much time is appropriate for each category is God's business once we have committed to his purpose.

unnecessary; all should be instruments of his will. We each need to hold our real life schedules up against this list to see if we presently allot appropriate time for each category.

Deciding how much time is appropriate for each category is God's business once we have committed to his purpose. The way we divide our time among the categories listed will be very much individualized for each of us because God has a different specific purpose for each of our lives. Some Christian doctors should be pouring themselves into the loving care of office patients ten to twelve hours a day, while others should be working with patients half-time and in mentoring ministry the other half. All of us should be very careful to give our family members the time they need, but that amount of time will vary depending on our family situations.

None of the categories listed above should be left off of any Christian doctor's list, but the proportionate time spent in each will be different for each of us.

How do we know how much time to spend in each important area of our lives? Let us suggest three guidelines:

1. **Be certain you are committed to God's foundational purpose** for the time in your life.
2. **Be deliberate.** If we let life shape our time, instead of deliberately organizing our time, Satan will shift our schedule according to his priorities.

When I was a medical missionary in Nigeria, I loved my work and poured myself into it, assuming that my wife would let me know if she needed more time. My wife has a sacrificial love for me. I only discovered that she needed more of me when it was too late to give it without sacrificing my life in missions.

–Al Weir, M.D.

3. **Be prayerful.** Pray to God on a weekly basis about each category and ask him to readjust your time in that category according to his will. It is our responsibility to want his will and his responsibility to make it clear.

A very helpful tool for your time-management tool kit is a prioritization system you can apply to the activities on your to-do list. You can use a simple three-part system like the following:

A. The activity is urgent and important to the successful performance of my job;
B. The activity is important but not urgent to the successful performance of my job;

C. The activity is urgent but not important to the successful performance of my job.

Let's define the terms. *Urgent* means that it must be accomplished today if it is to be done successfully. It has a deadline of today. *Important* means that if it is not accomplished, my job performance or goal achievement will be compromised. You will notice that there is no <u>D</u> category for items that are neither urgent nor important. Those activities don't belong anywhere on your work-related to-do list. If you must list them, put them to the side as reminders of "time fillers" if you ever have the luxury of unfilled time.

Those activities that are Priority <u>A</u> will include things that must be accomplished today and are vital to the achievement of your goals. Pre-scheduled patient appointments would be a prime example of A's, as would a staff meeting you are expected to lead. They are urgent (deadline of today) and important (to the successful performance of your job).

Activities in the <u>B</u> category will be just as important as A's, but will have a future deadline. They might include things like a meeting planned for next Tuesday, scheduling an appointment with your own personal physician for a non-urgent medical concern, or drafting a memo about a decision you need to make with your partners.

Tasks in the <u>C</u> category may have a sense of urgency about them – they need to be done today if they are going to be done – but they do not pass the importance test. An example of a C activity would be a Rotary Club meeting. If you're a member of Rotary, you're expected to attend weekly meetings. If that meeting is on Wednesday, it will show up on your to-do list for Wednesday. But is it vital to the successful performance of your job as a physician or dentist? You may be able to justify it as a public relations initiative of tangential benefit to your practice, but it can hardly be considered in the same category as patient care.

Now you are ready to apply the priorities to your to-do list. Be honest. Discern the difference between A's and C's. They will both feel urgent, but you must distinguish between "the tyranny of the urgent" and the "vital few." The deadlines will help you discern between the A's and the B's.

Once you have prioritized your planned activities, you can refine the list. First, eliminate as many C's as possible. If they aren't important, they don't belong on your list. Reduce the clutter of your mind by dismissing them. You may sense an immediate reduction of stress. If some of the C items still hold your interest, keep them available until you've made sure you have enough time to complete everything in your Priority A category.

The second step in refining your planned activities is to evaluate the potential for delegating the remaining items. Delegate those items that can

Delegate those items that can be accomplished better, quicker, or more cost-effectively by others.

Most people find a wealth of personal creativity when faced with the unhealthy and unrealistic facts about their time-usage habits.

be accomplished better, quicker, or more cost-effectively by others. You may want to delegate to subordinates, to colleagues, or even to superiors if that is an option, as long as it gets the job done better, quicker, or cheaper. Delegation may need to be negotiated, especially with colleagues or superiors, but if it makes sense to you to delegate, it may also make sense to them.

Third, take another look at all the activities within each priority, and give each item a sub-ranking to make sure you accomplish the most important items first. Your priority list might now have rankings of A-1, A-2, A-3, B-1, and so forth. Total up the projected time required to accomplish all your Priority A's. If it exceeds the time you have available in the day, you have a choice. You either have to delegate more, work longer that day, or find ways to accomplish the tasks in less than the projected time.

If your Priority A list always exceeds a reasonable amount of time for a workday, you are suffering a chronic marginless condition, and heading for serious physical, emotional, and spiritual pain. It is time for you to study *Margin.*[3]

Most people find a wealth of personal creativity when faced with the unhealthy and unrealistic facts about their time-usage habits. They re-evaluate their priorities, explore delegation alternatives, and uncover ideas to improve their efficiency.

A fourth refinement is to combine similar tasks within each priority. Combining computer tasks, for example, is more efficient than getting in and out of the computer at different times throughout the day. Combining meetings is also useful, especially if you are required to travel to another location like the hospital to attend them.

Managing Interruptions

Interruptions are normal phenomenas in everyone's work pattern. Family physicians who want to preserve continuity of care need to anticipate those patients who will present with urgent medical needs every day. The job of obstetricians is defined by expected interruptions. Dental emergencies are part of the routine for dentists. Some characteristics of interruptions can be anticipated and time can be allotted for them.

For example, primary care physicians can expect a daily demand for urgent care to be about 6 to 8 percent of their patient base. About six to eight patients per one hundred will present with an urgent need on any given weekday. Similar patterns can be measured in any other practice, and schedules can be adjusted to anticipate the interruptions by leaving time for them at the end of each morning and each afternoon schedule.

Interruptions can also be managed by having a back-up plan in place such as having patients seen by a mid-level practitioner or less-busy colleague. The ultimate back-up is the emergency department of your local hospital.

Identifying Your Prime Time

Some of us are morning people and others work better in the afternoon. Managing your time wisely involves knowing when you are most likely to do your best work, and structuring your schedule to preserve your prime time for your most important tasks. When you're tired, you're less likely to be efficient. Simple tasks can get bogged down and the risk for error increases. If you're fresh in the morning, try to complete your Priority A's before you reach your energy limit.

Celebrating Accomplishments

Make it your habit to cross off each task on your to-do list as you accomplish it. It's amazing how this simple act will affirm your sense of achievement. Physically seeing a list of completed assignments prompts celebration. It gives you a sense of being in control of your schedule rather than being a victim of it, and encourages you to extend your effectiveness by using the time management tools even more consistently.

When you complete your Priority A list ahead of your projections for the required time, reward yourself by moving ahead with a B item, having fun with a C activity, or just taking some time off for yourself.

Refine Your Projections

Reexamine your projected time requirements after you have completed the tasks on your daily to-do list. If an item took more time than you projected, consider how it may have gotten more complex than you anticipated and think about how it could have been accomplished more efficiently. If you completed an item in less time than you expected, celebrate the fact and make a mental note for the next time you have to accomplish a similar task.

Efficient Meetings

Meetings are the bane of our modern society. They are notoriously inefficient, but still essential for communication, which is the lifeblood of organizations. The next time you are in a meeting, do a mental calculation of the hourly rates of the people sitting around the table. Multiply the total by the number of hours of the meeting, and you may be astonished at the

Make it your habit to cross off each task on your to-do list as you accomplish it. It's amazing how this simple act will affirm your sense of achievement.

Wise leadership involves constantly discerning the shifting priorities of agenda items within the real constraints of time.

cost of the event. Then compare the cost to the value of the outcome. Brace yourself for a sobering conclusion.

Time management techniques as described in this chapter are designed to improve personal productivity, but they can also be applied to achieve more efficient meetings. An agenda can do for a meeting what a to-do list can do for an individual. It outlines the plan for how time will be spent. It articulates what is expected to be accomplished in a selected period of time. Individuals accomplish tasks; meetings accomplish decisions.

If a meeting is scheduled without an agenda, the result can be as unpredictable and inefficient as if an individual starts a day without plans or ambitions. Productive meetings begin with an agenda that the leader of the group constructed with forethought. An agenda represents respect for the time and energy of everyone who will attend the meeting.

Wise leaders will also consider alternative methods for communication other than meetings, just as individuals will look for options to delegate tasks. Meeting time is precious and should be reserved for those issues that require face-to-face dialogue, consensus, and joint decisions.

Other types of communication should be kept off the time-limited meeting agenda, and left for newsletters, e-mail, voice mail, posters, or other less costly methods. Likewise, determine who really needs to be at the meeting, and who should stay behind to use their time more effectively.

Finally, set time-limited expectations for each discussion item. Wise leaders recognize the need for some flexibility here, but it is important to pace the agenda realistically.

It is dangerous to try cramming a discussion that requires two hours into a twenty-minute time slot. The decision that comes out of a compromised discussion has little chance of succeeding. Those who weren't given a voice will have a hard time supporting the decision, even if they granted their vote for the sake of time.

If the discussion is allowed to ramble, the rest of the agenda may suffer – and timely decisions on important issues along with it.

Wise leadership involves constantly discerning the shifting priorities of agenda items within the real constraints of time.

Teach Others Time Management

If the time management techniques are helpful to you, consider sharing them with your colleagues and staff. You will help each of them manage their own lives, increase the productivity of your entire practice, and establish a common language to hold each other accountable.

Simplify

Sometimes there is just too much to cram into each day. Then we are either forced to do things too quickly, resulting in poor performance, or forced to leave out activities we had planned. Cramming is how we usually handle it, with canceling as our escape valve. We see patient after patient with life-changing problems where we only take care of the technical issues, ignoring the more important social, emotional, and spiritual ones. We just don't have the time to spend with them. Week after week we plan to get to this conference or that ball game until the time pressure builds up so much at the last minute that we cancel those plans. Many of us live the same kind of lives. Often our families suffer the most.

If this is the way we are living, we need to simplify our lives. We need to decrease the number of activities we try to accomplish each day. How do we decide what to drop? Dawn Reno in her book *The Unofficial Guide to Managing Time* suggests we look at the activities that fill our schedule and divide them into three categories:

> *There are some activities that are harmful to the important activities in our lives. We should identify them and drop them.*

- •Those you can't live without;
- •Those that are important;
- •Those that you wouldn't miss [that are not important].

Perhaps we should add a fourth:
- •Those that interfere with the important.

Then we should make some choices, moving from the bottom of the list up. There are some activities that are harmful to the important activities in our lives. We should identify those and drop them. These may be sinful or innocuous or even good in themselves, but if they prevent us from moving toward our foundational purpose in life through important activities, they should be reduced or eliminated.

Those inhibitory or harmful activities will be different for each of us and may include recreational time, hobbies, a second job, or even church communities. Examine your life, cut out the inhibitory or harmful, and then cut out some of the third category—those that you wouldn't miss.

Dick Swenson, in his book, *Margin*, says it is better for us to have some margin in our lives to allow for the unexpected important than it is to pack our lives with extra activities of little importance.

It physically hurts me when I am rushing so fast through my patient schedule that I can't relax for five minutes when my father steps over from his office to see me. I need to reorder the time before my office practice, the time after my office

Learning new habits often challenges us to re-think old habits. Learning time management requires us to confront the beliefs that have defined our work patterns in the past.

practice, and the number of patients I see within that practice so that I can spend five minutes communicating with the greatest man I know if he should happen to pop in to visit. There are less important things on my agenda that I really wouldn't miss if I just cut them out of my schedule.

—Al Weir, M.D.

Learning new habits often challenges us to rethink old habits. Learning time management requires us to confront the beliefs that have defined our work patterns in the past. This process is good, although it can be painful. I believe this kind of introspection is particularly beneficial for Christian physicians and dentists who are committed to honoring the Lord with their time. Sometimes it may be difficult for a practice to assess its own needs in time management, patient flow, and scheduling problems. Practice consultants, if chosen wisely, may be worth their cost in the long run, to settle these problems in ways that are both cost-efficient and comfortable for patients.

The crucial issue is to remember that the management tools described here are resources. They are formats and concepts, but their real value is only discovered in the disciplined and consistent application of these tools. The implications for Christian physicians and dentists who use these tools are wide-ranging. They have practical value by extending your efficiency and effectiveness at work. And they have eternal value in challenging us all to establish God-honoring priorities.

THREE QUESTIONS TO ASK YOURSELF
1. Upon what foundational principle do I plan all of my activities?
2. What activities can I remove from my schedule to allow more time for the important?
3. What one responsibility can I delegate to another that will allow me more time to spend doing that which only I can do?

THREE ACTIONS TO CONSIDER
1. List the categories of activities in your life that you believe God wishes you to accomplish.
2. Make a chart of this week's activities and categorize them by their importance and urgency.
3. Ask God to show you an accountability partner with whom you could meet monthly to pray with and review your time utilization.

PRAYER

Dear God,

Thank you for the gift and responsibility of time. Show me how to use it wisely. Let me not waste the instrument that you have placed in my hands to redeem a lost world. Let me care for those who need care. Let me trust you to achieve your goals with my life. Grant me the discipline I need to fashion a schedule that will honor you.

–Amen

NOTES:

1. Swenson, Richard A., *Margin*, NavPress, 1992.
2. For more on polarities, see *www.polaritymanagement.com*.
3. Swenson, ibid.

CHAPTER 11

Managing Money

*S*everal years ago two Christian colleagues sat comparing notes during a lull *in the proceedings of a missions conference. Both were in their seventies, still actively practicing medicine, one a general surgeon and the other a family practitioner. Both were eager to retire and "do missions," but neither was able to do so because continued practice was necessary for their financial security. The surgeon's pension fund amounted to "less than $150,000" and the other admitted to something even less. These were successful doctors through whose hands a fortune had passed; yet, both stated that they were "working because I have to."*

Even more tragic, both of these colleagues had once heard a call from God into missions and could not follow that call because they were bound by their finances. Nor was it likely that either of them would ever be able to engage in the generous giving to ministries that they were obviously interested in. Two of the most satisfying and productive disciplines of the Christian life, service in missions and joyful giving, would likely forever remain beyond the reach of these two doctors.

How does this happen? How can a person in the top 5 percent of wage earners in the United States practice his profession for a lifetime and anticipate retirement on a low income? How can God's people hear God's call and find it impossible to follow? How can you keep this from happening to you? The following simple and basic preventive measures may keep your life free to follow God's call: having a biblical view of money and material things; having a plan for the allocation and spending of money; maintaining an aversion to debt—all the while controlling excessive consumption.

A BIBLICAL VIEW OF MONEY AND MATERIAL THINGS

A fourth-year medical student with an unrestricted credit line used educational loans to buy an expensive automobile. When questioned about her motive, she replied, "I figure I owe it to myself to go with what turns me

Our responsibility as followers of Jesus is to understand the implications of God's ownership and incorporate them into our attitudes and practices concerning money.

on." She bought a car that cost three times more than a brand-new entry level sedan. She was looking for transportation—and self-gratification.

The Bible clearly teaches, most notably in the parable of the stewards (or the talents) that God owns all material things (Matt. 25:14-30). He has created everything and he has a right to it. He owns all the silver and all the gold (Hag. 2:8). All that we have, whether we have worked hard for it or not, was entrusted to us for his great purposes. We can take nothing with us when we leave this life. Our responsibility as followers of Jesus is to understand the implications of God's ownership and incorporate them into our attitudes and practices concerning money.

In his parable of the talents, Jesus tells us to actively manage that which God has placed in our care so as to earn his commendation: "Well done, good and faithful servant." The steward who did not actively manage was called "wicked and lazy," and was cast into darkness. These words place on the Christian the responsibility to do things differently than our impulses, appetites, and competitive relationships would suggest.

Doctors are just ordinary men and women when it comes to following our natural impulses. A young surgeon was explaining why she had spent so much money on very luxurious living room furniture. She gave several reasonable advantages, such as long wear and enduring style, but finally added, "Let's face it. I just like nice things!"

The habitual consumption of material things, many of which are bought on impulse, results in the kind of spending and financial imprisonment suffered by the physicians mentioned in the beginning of this chapter. Awareness of divine ownership and a strong sense of careful, responsible stewardship will override an excessive appetite for material things and leave us free to serve when our Master calls.

The goal of biblical financial stewardship is not to hoard wealth, or to spend it to satisfy our own appetites, but to use it wisely for God's glory and God's redemptive purpose. Storing up wealth for its own sake, or to achieve the illusion of a secure future, is dangerous and misguided (Luke 12:13-21; 1 Tim. 6:9-10, 17). Investing for eternity involves giving generously, being "rich in good deeds," "rich toward God," and growing the kingdom of God on earth (1 Tim. 6:18-19, Luke 12:21, Luke 16:9). It takes both self-denial and an open hand to use money for these purposes.

Living simply and saving are important biblical principles, but they are not ends in themselves. We live simply in order to temper the love of money and material things that can crowd God out of our lives, preventing us from becoming spiritually mature (Luke 8:14). We save so that we will be free to follow God's direction with our time and resources in the future. Although we may hope to retire from our profession, we will never retire from Christian service.

It is not enough to be "above it all" and act as though money management is a crass and unspiritual pursuit. Our money should be a hammer in the mighty hand of God. The Bible instructs us as Christians to be good stewards, to give, and to serve following the example of Jesus Christ (Mark 10:45). The penalty for poor stewardship is severe (Matt. 5:29).

Jesus and other biblical writers identify six ways to honor God with our wealth:

1. Our money honors God when we use it to care for our families: "If anyone does not provide for his relatives, and especially for his immediate family, he has denied the faith and is worse than an unbeliever" (1 Tim 5:8).

2. Our money honors God when we give to the poor and needy: "You still lack one thing. Sell everything you have and give to the poor and you will have treasure in heaven. Then come, follow me" (Luke 18:22).

3. Our money honors God when used to support the church and its work of redeeming the world: "And he sat down opposite the treasury, and watched the multitude putting money into the treasury. Many rich people put in large sums. And a poor widow came, and put in two copper coins, which make a penny. And he called his disciples to him and said to them, 'Truly, I say to you, this poor widow has put in more than all of those who are contributing to the treasury. For they all contributed out of their abundance; but she out of her poverty has put in everything that she had, her whole living" (Mark 12:41-44, RSV).

4. Our money honors God when used to fulfill our civic responsibility: "Render therefore to Caesar the things that are Caesar's, and to God the things that are God's" (Matt. 22:21, RSV).

5. Our money honors God when we enjoy life with it according to his biblical guidelines: "Behold, what I have seen to be good and to be fitting is to eat and drink and find enjoyment in all the toil with which one toils under the sun the few days of his life that God has given him, for this is his lot. Every man also to whom God has given wealth and possessions and power to enjoy them, and to accept his lot and find enjoyment in his toil–this is the gift of God" (Eccl. 5:18-19, RSV).

6. Our money honors God when we pour it out as an act of love for Jesus: "And while he was at Bethany in the house of Simon the leper, as he sat at table, a woman came with an alabaster jar of ointment of pure nard, very costly, and she broke the jar and poured it over his head. But there were

It is not enough to be "above it all" and act as though money management is a crass and unspiritual pursuit. Our money should be a hammer in the mighty hand of God.

*We, more
than most,
have been
blessed with
money
and the
tremendous
opportunity
it gives
(when placed
in God's
hands) to
bring a lost
world back
into his arms.*

some who said to themselves indignantly, 'Why was the ointment thus wasted? For this ointment might have been sold for more than three hundred denarii, and given to the poor.' And they reproached her. But Jesus said, 'Let her alone; why do you trouble her? She has done a beautiful thing to me'" (Mark 14:3-9, RSV).

God cares about our money because he cares about our hearts: "For where your treasure is, there your heart will be also" (Matt. 6:21). As doctors, we, more than most, have been blessed with money and the pleasure it brings. We, more than most, have been blessed with money and the danger it brings. We, more than most, have been blessed with money and the tremendous opportunity it gives (when placed in God's hands) to bring a lost world back into his arms.

A FINANCIAL CONTROL PLAN

One cannot be a good steward (a good manager of that which belongs to someone else) without developing a weekly, monthly, or annual plan to deal responsibly with the money that God provides for our use.

A financial control plan consists of three parts: an **income component, an allocation component,** and **a spending component.** Following such a plan should make us aware of exactly where we stand financially, without being obsessed with money. This financial awareness is critical both in allowing us to avoid debt and in freeing us to give when God calls. Unfortunately, many of us drift through our practice lives with the hope that the money is enough; but we live with the fear that it is not and with the true awareness of very little about money matters.

At financial management seminars, when those attending are told that they should know the balance in their checkbook within ten to twenty dollars, a giggle or snicker usually circulates through the audience. Many just don't get it.

Income

Many doctors these days are salaried and can predict with a high degree of accuracy how much money will be coming into the household. We also have significant input as to what kind of income we will seek in our future. One of the basic questions that must be considered along the way is, "How much is enough?" The stock answer to this question is: "Enough to give on, live on, and pay taxes on." There is considerable personal preference and subjectivity in these answers, but once answered, they become your goal for your income production.

This question really should be asked by two sets of doctors. The first set would be doctors early in their careers. Doctors starting out have the opportunity to set a limit and live within that limit without becoming covered up by layers of wealth. Before we acquire a lifestyle that sticks like tar to our hearts, we have the chance to define our lifestyle and plan the rest of our income to be spent on God's work. Or we can plan to use more of our time without remuneration for his service, for example, in providing free or low-cost care to the poor or underserved, or those in full-time Christian service.

One doctor starting out did it this way:

When we transitioned to private practice, our income rose sharply. At first we were only intentional about continuing to tithe, giving 10 percent to our local church. However, our desire to give to a variety of different causes, and now having the means to give more, resulted in us giving well beyond 10 percent that first year. We became aware of this when we prepared our taxes for that year. Not only did we have the joy of giving throughout the year, we had an additional sense of satisfaction as we reviewed the yearly totals. That's when we became more intentional about giving. With few exceptions, we narrowed our giving to only those efforts that in some way furthered the kingdom or obeyed the commandments to attend to the needs of the poor, widows, orphans, etc. We purposed each year to give more the next year —"more" meaning a higher percentage of our income. That usually meant more in total giving — but not every year. We eventually leveled out at 40 percent of our gross income. It was very easy for us to live on the remaining. We kept our standard of living at a level consistent with the money that was left over after giving and savings. And we lived happily and comfortably. I truly believe God's blessing was the major part of that result. I know he put the joy and satisfaction in our hearts. And I suspect he positively intervened in our economics in ways we did not know.

—A Christian doctor

Many of us, though, have developed an income and lifestyle that is far more extravagant than that which pleases God. If this is true for you, how do you get back to an income and lifestyle that would make God smile?

If you are early in your career, now is the time to honor God by setting limits on your future income and lifestyle. Many of us, though, have developed an income and lifestyle that is far more extravagant than that which pleases God. If this is true for you, how do you get back to an income and lifestyle that would make God smile? There are only two steps that can get us there: putting on the brakes, and giving.

If you've already developed a lifestyle that has or will lead to debt or to inadequate funds for retirement and inadequate resources for biblical giving, consulting a financial counselor might be very helpful. Time in prayer with your spouse examining your purpose in life is likely to be important. Developing well defined spending guidelines and establishing "speed bumps" for impulsive spending will also help.

Certainly God has a plan or a counselor with a plan toward godly stewardship for each of us. You cannot pretend to be a follower of Christ if you are driven by your money.

They had reached the age of fifty with their kids nearly out of the home. They looked at their lives and realized that too much money was spent impulsively and selfishly. But how do you stop a three-decade habit of spending? Two sets of brakes were applied. The first was a fairly simple method of accountability with each other. Any time either was contemplating spending over two hundred dollars, he/she would have to call the spouse for permission. That certainly helped with individual impulse. Jewelry store and outdoor store expenditures fell.

But such a simple plan did not really help with the big desires that they fell into together. As they prayed for guidance, God laid out an additional plan. They decided to define the big extras in life as luxuries. The new hot tub, an addition on the house, a house at the lake, a ski boat, etc. would fit into the category of luxury. Anytime they chose to spend money on a luxury, they could do so, but would have to give an equal amount above the tithe to God's work. Such a plan served two purposes: first, any luxury would cost them twice as much, so they would have to think hard about the value of that luxury; secondly, if luxuries were chosen, God's work would be equally blessed.

The system was tested and has been successful. When they decided to build a new home, they committed to spending no more than the value of the house they owned, or to paying to God's work the equivalence of the difference. The architect promised them a house at their price. Three months of joyful planning with the architect brought them to a beautiful dream home. Then the builders came in with costs of $300,000 above the cost they had committed to. The doctor and his wife left the drawings on the architect's table and settled back into the good home that God had already given them, expanded a room for $30,000 and gave an equal amount to help CMDA set up its media center.

They could easily have afforded the notes for the new house, but not the extra hundreds of thousands of dollars that would have been required to honor their commitment to the Lord. Though they had lost a dream home, the couple felt nothing but joy.

On the other hand, they also felt joyful as a family spending time at their lake house in the summer; and as they settled without guilt into that pleasure, they gave an amount equal to the yearly cost of their lake house to the Lord's work, and as a result, a young Christian girl in Albania received $10,000 a year toward her education and a poor single mom got a new roof for her house.

This couple found a way to put the brakes on their own spending at the same time they increased their giving. This type of plan might work for you. Certainly God has a plan or a counselor with a plan toward godly stewardship for each of us.

You cannot pretend to be a follower of Christ if you are driven by your money.

Allocation

An allocation plan places limits on future spending. In order to plan properly, you might collect a financial history from three periods during the preceding year to provide a representative schedule of expenditures that is corrected for seasonal variations. This can be done from the register in your checkbook, or by using home financial software tools such as Quicken™ or Microsoft Money™. The plan is then based on your past record, being as frugal as possible, but with enough leeway so that you do not chafe under the discipline.

Each spending category should receive its proper allocation: giving, taxes, housing, utilities, food, automobile and other transportation, medical and dental expenses, entertainment, vacations, etc. The amount allocated to each category may need to be adjusted in order to meet your financial goals. Once the plan is developed, it can provide boundaries that will help restrain impulse buying – the vulnerable point of any financial control plan.

The actual writing of the checks or arranging direct electronic transfer of funds from a bank account should be undertaken by the person in the household most adept at handling finances. Items that are not allocated should not be purchased unless some other purchase is denied. Every violation of the financial control plan should be reviewed and corrected for the long term. A plan is only as good as the care taken to adhere to it.

The actual writing of the checks or arranging direct electronic transfer of funds from a bank account should be undertaken by the person in the household most adept at handling finances.

A medical student, called by God to the mission field, had acquired $128,000 in debt, a sum that would have prevented his responding to that call. He had heard of Project MedSend and received the counsel that his loans could be paid off by MedSend as he served on the field after his three-year residency. With counsel from the MedSend staff, a plan for repayment of the interest on his debt (and some of the principal) was agreed upon for his residency years, when his salary would be about $44,000 annually.

At the halfway point of his residency, the physician contacted project MedSend to apply for the expected loan repayment grant. However, he had not implemented the sound and reasonable plan he had committed to and his indebtedness had risen to $143,000! The resident almost lost his opportunity for missions because of his lack of financial discipline. With God's help and Project MedSend's guidance, he reassessed his situation and applied the necessary financial discipline. This allowed him to repay in excess of $16,000 annually until he left for the mission field, thereby complying with the terms of his grant and stepping onto the path where God had led him.

Perhaps with such an encounter early in his career, this young doctor will learn what many of us older doctors have never learned: All of the plans in the world will not control our finances unless we have the discipline to follow the plans. Project MedSend provided this young man with accountability. Many of us would be wise to program accountability into our financial planning, with our spouses, with a mentor, or with a financial planner we trust.

GUIDELINES FOR ALLOCATING INCOME

The question is frequently asked, "Should I spend with some order of priorities? The answer, of course, is "Yes." Here is one biblically-based priority sequence of allocating income that works very well:

1. Giving
2. Taxes
3. Debt repayment
4. Savings
5. Living

Giving is what God does. Giving is what we, too, must do if we wish to become the people he created us to be. Those who have placed giving to God as the highest priority for their spending will uniformly affirm the blessing that results. But perhaps you wonder: How much should I give? Should I give before or after taxes? Should I give 10 percent or is that just legalism from Old Testament times? Should I give to the local church or should I support ministries that are not highly visible and popular?

You can't go wrong if your giving is based on your gross earnings, that is, before taxes. You can't go wrong if you use 10 percent (the tithe) as the base, and think of giving as that which comes after the tithe. You can't go wrong if you support your local church and also give where God is working outside your local church.

Years ago, a student in Texas heard a talk on financial management that included a discussion on giving. The speaker said, "It's okay to go beyond the 10 percent goal in giving. In fact, as an expression of gratitude to God and the joy of giving, some might feel compelled to give 30 percent or 50 percent or 60 percent to the Lord's work."

Years later, that student met the conference speaker in another part of the country and told him, "When you suggested that it was okay to go beyond 10 percent, it opened a new door for me. Since then, I have practiced incremental increases in my giving, in spite of my growing family and growing financial pressures. My experience has been that the Lord provides and that the discipline required has brought satisfaction rather than frustration. Giving first keeps everything that remains in order."

Doctors who really grasp God's understanding of money often seek to systematize their giving so that it can be consistent:

As we entered our fifties and sent our kids off to their own lives, we realized that our money could be a valuable instrument for God's service. We could now more easily direct it toward his work. Though we still had some educational responsibilities, those would taper off over the years. My wife and I committed to steadily increasing our giving over the next ten years from the usual 10 percent, by 1 percent a year, until we reached a consistent 20 percent yearly gift to God's work and the care of the poor. It does take a letting go of control over our future security and we do feel a bit of loss as we hand it over to the Lord, but we trust God to use the funds for his purposes and are content with that.

—*A Christian doctor*

Some doctors gauge the amount of their gift by whether the gift is large enough to hurt.

Some doctors gauge the amount of their gift by whether the gift is large enough to hurt. One doctor discovered that even that gauge may be short-changing our Lord:

When the campaign began to raise funds for God's work through CMDA, we felt that we should contribute, so we made our pledge. As the campaign continued, we felt that our gift was not large enough, so we pledged a bit more—enough to hurt a bit. God continued to speak to us and we raised our pledge again and it hurt more. But God didn't stop there. God continued to work on our hearts; we knew that he wanted more from us, so we made the largest pledge to the Lord's work that we had ever made. It was certainly more than we could afford. And, do you know what? It began to feel good!

—*A Christian doctor*

Taxes are inevitable. They must be paid, and prompt payment of taxes not only renders unto Caesar the things that belong to Caesar, but also keeps you out of trouble.

A two-income physician family was two years behind in the payment of their taxes. This delinquency in their financial responsibility placed a profound strain on their marriage. The interest and penalties they constantly had to pay kept them feeling "tight for cash," and was magnified by their inability to curb their appetite for consumer frills. The wealth that had been available to free them for joyful living had wrapped itself around them and was smothering them because they had not accepted the responsibility of the taxes that comes with the privilege of income.

Debt repayment will also prevent you from being a slave to your lenders (Prov. 22:7). One should always try to exceed the "minimum monthly pay-

*In a
society
that runs
on debt and
consumption,
it seems
paradoxical
to work hard
and then to
have to use
restraint in
spending
that which
has been
earned.*

ment," or "minimum payment due"–devices designed to enrich the lender. Any discretionary funds available should be used to pay down debt. A desirable goal for every Christian is to be debt-free.

Savings should be habitually implemented as a healthy financial practice and it should be taught to your children. If even a small percentage of income is saved, substantial gains can accumulate when saving becomes a habit that starts early in one's career. Forcing oneself to save through pension plan contributions may be sufficient for retirement security, and the saving that is done additionally can be thought of as "saving up" for non-allocated items, gifts, and other discretionary uses that may not be allocated already.

Living expenditures must be managed from what is left, and here is the rub. A disciplined financial manager will not buy things that he or she cannot afford to buy. In a society that runs on debt and consumption, it seems paradoxical to work hard and then have to use restraint in spending that which has been earned. But short-term self-denial pays big dividends in providing financial security, freedom from money obsessions, debt-free living, freedom to give to God, and joyful service to him.

Becoming and Remaining Debt Free

Once we have controlled our spending and planned our giving, we must deal with any debt that we have accumulated. To live debt-free should be the goal of the Christian. The Bible reminds us that indebtedness is a form of slavery (Prov. 22:7). Debt must be repaid. The worst kind of debt is unsecured debt, where there is no asset that can be sold to repay it. This is usually consumer debt, credit card debt. When the full amount of the credit is not paid each month, the item purchased may be used up, broken, or worn out before it is paid for. Several principles can be used as a guide to becoming and remaining debt free:

1. Develop a financial plan with a proper priority list and execute that plan, practicing a schedule of giving that is guided by your interaction with God.
2. Eliminate credit card and consumer debt. Pay off the highest interest indebtedness first and pay ahead on the principal of any loans when it is possible.
3. Develop a sense of stewardship that will override any longing to have what others seem to enjoy. Achieve your sense of self-worth from who you are in God's economy rather than from what you own (and the label it carries). Competition in consumption is an effective tool of the advertising media. Don't be seduced!

4. Develop a healthy respect for the dangers inherent in the credit card. If you cannot control your use of credit cards, cut them up and apply for a debit card, which will warn you of overspending. Even paying the full balance every month, you will spend more with a credit card because it is convenient.

5. Try to buy only what you need, rather than everything you want. Delay purchases over a certain threshold (a hundred dollars, for example) for a week or a month as a "cooling-off period." Many have testified that with time they have forgotten the appeal of something they "just loved and couldn't live without!"

6. Shop with a list and buy only what is on the list. If something has not been listed, put it on the following week's list.

7. Don't "go shopping." Shopping is the great American indoor sport in which people who already have everything look for things to buy that they don't need. Stay at home and read a good book–maybe the Good Book!

Achieve your sense of self-worth from who you are in God's economy rather than from what you own (and the label it carries).

Once you are out of debt, the same principles will keep you out of debt. A financial control plan is not a straightjacket. It is liberating, because it promotes instant awareness of your real financial condition. For the Christian, it is especially liberating since it allows biblical giving and biblical service.

A young married couple, heady with the fruits of a young practice, began to analyze their financial situation after a financial seminar at the CMDA annual convention. "We realized that we were spending more in monthly interest on our 'Doctor House' than it cost to send our two children to a private school for a year," they said.

How did they come to buy such an expensive home? They went along with everything the builder suggested and he convinced them that they needed the best such as a $15,000 stainless steel refrigerator with a famous designer's logo prominently displayed on the door.

"We sold the house (having to wait for another doctor to come along and buy it) and with the equity, paid cash for a very nice home in a neighborhood with a better school system to which we sent our children."

The nicest part of this story was the point they found most satisfying:

"We had always wanted to give and to serve in our church and on the mission field. We have been liberated to do both."

It is difficult for Christians to fully adopt a view of the world that is radically different from the secular, post-Christian, post-modern world in which we live.

The bottom line is, most of us can manage our own finances with a little discipline, about an hour a month of study, a tax attorney to help us take advantage of any laws that will allow us to reduce our taxes, and a periodic checkup by a financial counselor or Christian financial management firm that does not sell an investment product.

A tax attorney will keep you abreast of changes in the tax laws as they relate to incorporated practices, pension plan regulations, and the "must" for busy people who tend to procrastinate: a will and the legal documents related to an estate plan. A Christian attorney does not come with a halo or as a sanctified oracle. However, a Christian attorney will be much more likely to respect your wishes regarding charitable giving from your estate and can suggest various trust instruments that will allow you to increase your giving, leave more for your heirs, and dramatically reduce estate taxes.

Christian financial planners can be of real help to Christian doctors who choose not to take the time to try to do it all themselves. Remember that the word "Christian" may be a form of advertisement rather than a sign of a Spirit-filled life. Be certain the person you choose to be your counselor is well referenced by people you trust. Competence is also critical.

Finding a true Christian financial counselor is best because he or she will best understand your motivation for saving and giving. A competent and honest non-Christian financial counselor may also honor your responsibility before God to use his money well, but self-interest is difficult to eliminate in anyone you choose to help you.

Some Christian foundations are very sound in this area. They advise and can suggest products such as donor-directed trusts that allow one to give, yet accumulate money for larger gifts to be given in a later year. They charge a fee for their advice, but do not burden the client with sales pressure.

IT'S HOW YOU LOOK AT THINGS

It is difficult for Christians to fully adopt a view of the world that is radically different from the secular, post-Christian, post-modern world in which we live. We feel it is our right to have whatever anyone else has and to be able to do what anyone else does. We have worked hard for whatever we have accumulated and feel we deserve some pleasurable rewards.

The problem with this thinking is that it is not biblical. The rich man who retired, put up his feet, and took his ease was not called a fool because there is anything wrong with retirement or with being a successful businessman who needs a bigger warehouse. Jesus put his finger squarely on the man's problem: He had left God out of the equation. He had stored up things for himself and was not rich toward God. The part of this story that stings us most is Jesus' statement that it will be thus for anyone with the same worldview! (Luke 12:16-21).

A secular view of the world denies absolutes, and puts its hope in pleasure and treasure. Jesus calls his followers to a life of sacrifice and service and to lay up treasures in heaven where it will not become moth-eaten, rusted-out, or stolen. Our money is to be used here for God's redemptive purposes. It has often been said, that you can't take it with you, but you can send it on ahead.

The secularist, pondering the great questions of life, is confounded by the questions: "Where did I come from?" "Why am I here?" and "Where am I going?"

The Christian answers these questions: "I am created in the image of God; I am here to glorify God and enjoy him forever; and, I am going to the place that the resurrected Christ has prepared for me. I do not have to compete on the world's terms. What matters most is that I am obedient to Christ and can revel in what he has done for me. Material things are not a valid measure of success, and it is not true that 'he who finishes with the most toys, wins.'"

The old rhyme has it right: "Only one life, 'twill soon be past. Only what's done for Christ will last." If we as serious Christians believed and practiced this world view, we would not have problems with stewardship of what God has placed in our care.

Jesus calls his followers to a life of sacrifice and service and to lay up treasures in heaven where it will not become moth-eaten, rusted-out, or stolen.

GUIDELINES FOR SPENDING

How you spend your money after you pay taxes is one of the most critical decisions you will make in your personal financial planning. Living within your means and not trying to keep up with your colleagues is one of the fundamental principles of financial freedom. You should develop a budget and stick to it. According to Stanley and Danko, authors of *The Millionaire Next Door*, physicians do not tend to be wealth accumulators. Their research found that among all major high income-producing occupations, physicians have a significantly low propensity to accumulate wealth. One of the benefits of financial planning is that this process allows you to see how you are spending your money and understand the implications your spending patterns have on your current and long-term financial well being. In other words, you can decide if current consumption outweighs the benefits of a more secure retirement or earlier financial independence.

Home Mortgage

The biggest expense for most doctors is their mortgage. As a general rule you should keep your mortgage payment (including taxes and insurance) at 28 to 35 percent of your pre-tax income. You should usually also pay a down payment of 20 percent of the purchase price to avoid expensive personal mortgage insurance. In certain situations, the lender will waive the

It will take approximately 368 months for them to pay off the original $10,000 balance. Over this time period, they will also pay $9,696 in interest charges.

personal mortgage insurance if you are not able to come up with the 20 percent down payment.

Credit Cards

Credit cards are very convenient tools; however, if you are unable to pay your monthly charges in full you should not use them. Credit card debt is very expensive. For example, Dr. & Mrs. Smith have a balance of $10,000 in credit card debt. The credit card company is charging them 12 percent annual interest. The Smith's choose to pay only the minimum payment each month. It will take approximately 368 months for them to pay off the original $10,000 balance. Over this time period, they will also pay $9,696 in interest charges.

Investment Guidelines

As we have all witnessed, making money in the stock market is not as easy as it seemed during the 1990s. As a doctor, you have spent countless hours learning to be the very best at treating patients you can be. Unfortunately, most doctors no longer have the time to learn the basics of investing.

Essentially, you have two choices as to how you direct your dollars for investment. You can either be a loaner or an owner. You can loan your money to a bank, (i.e., buy a certificate of deposit); to the United States government, (i.e., buy a Treasury bond); or to corporations, (i.e., buy a corporate bond or shares of a bond mutual fund). Otherwise, you can be an owner, through buying individual stocks or shares of a stock mutual fund.

The main objective in choosing investments is to create a broadly diversified portfolio, which includes various types of investments that work well together as a team. History has shown owners make more money than loaners; in other words, the stock market has generally outperformed the bond market. However, it is prudent to include a bond allocation in your portfolio.

It's the offense of a team that sells tickets to football games, but it's the defense that wins the game. The same concept applies to your portfolio. Bonds (or loaned dollars) are the defense and help preserve value in declining stock markets. The empirical evidence shows bonds lag stocks because they have less risk. The performance of the entire portfolio should be your gauge rather than the individual components. The true benefits of diversification shine during volatile markets. The portfolio as a whole is safer than the individual investments.

There is no magic for accumulating wealth. It requires discipline to set aside money on a consistent basis. You must allow ample time for the money to grow. Emotions such as fear and greed are tough to handle; yet, you must separate your money from your emotions and remain committed to your investment strategy. Your money needs to grow in order to meet funding goals such as college and retirement or financial independence. The sooner you start investing for these goals the less you have to save for the desired result.

Investment Products

It is not possible in limited space to explain the variety of ways in which one can invest, but here are a few basics:

Common Stocks are shares in a company that give one the rights of ownership such as voting at the company's annual meeting. A company that distributes its profits does so in proportion to the number of shares owned by the shareholder.

Pros: Potential for high return, company ownership, historically proven winner.

Cons: Volatility; can lose entire investment.

Bonds are I.O.U.s or promissory notes of a corporation or municipality on which the owner receives a specific rate of interest and payment in full of the face value of the bond at a specified date of maturity. Because bonds produce income to the owner of the bond (interest) and interest is paid from company earnings, bonds are considered to be a less risky investment than stocks, which are not guaranteed to distribute company profits in the form of dividends. Bond values do fluctuate based on movements in interest rates, however.

Pros: Stable income stream, provides portfolio stability, Federal bonds are backed by the U.S. Government.

Cons: Low returns.

Mutual Funds are investment companies that use capital to buy shares of other companies, and then sell shares in itself to investors. A mutual fund may own shares in many different companies, thus providing diversification of investment as protection against the decline of a certain stock or industry. If the investment company charges a percentage fee to buy its shares, it is called a load fund. If it charges no sales fees, it is called a no-load fund.

Pros: Professional management, broad diversification, can be an inexpensive method of investing.

Cons: No control over capital gains and dividend distributions, lack of timely information on fund companies and their buy/sell movements, can lose entire investment.

There is no magic for accumulating wealth. It requires discipline to set aside money on a consistent basis.

The successful practitioner does not need to continue earning money that he or she could never spend, money that might be squandered by heirs.

A **certificate of deposit (CD)** is a savings account, usually in a bank, with a specified maturity date, on which that bank pays a fixed rate of interest. For example, a five-year CD at 6 percent will yield an income of 6 percent with interest compounding daily for five years. The Federal Deposit Insurance Corporation (FDIC) insures most bank CDs up to $100,000.

Pros: Safety of principal, FDIC insurance.

Cons: Returns after taxes and after inflation are very low.

An **annuity** is an investment instrument in which an individual pays an insurance company a specified capital sum in exchange for the promise by the insurer to pay monthly or quarterly payments, usually for the lifetime of the insured and sometimes for the lifetime of a surviving spouse as well. At the death of the survivor the remainder of the annuity usually reverts to the insurance company. There are many types of annuities, one of which, the charitable annuity, provides a charitable deduction in the year it is purchased.

Pros: Funds accumulate tax-deferred, death benefit option, can avoid probate by beneficiary designation.

Cons: High expenses and commissions.

A **broker** is an agent who handles orders to buy and sell the items listed above. For this the broker receives a fee. Discount brokers charge very low fees. Once a brokerage account is established, many transactions may be accomplished without any contact with the broker, via the Internet.

Pros: Brokers can provide good stock research and advice, discount brokerage provides an inexpensive investing alternative.

Cons: Buy/Sell pressure, brokers can provide bad advice, brokerage houses are commission-based operations, discount brokerages are impersonal with low level of service.

GUIDELINES FOR COLLEGE PLANNING

Most doctors want to provide at least four years of college for each of their children. There are various ways to save and no one method is best for everyone. The best method for you depends on your individual circumstances. Many doctors prefer a regular monthly investment method of accumulating funds for college. A direct draft from a designated account is an easy way to put these funds aside. It invests the money before you have a chance to spend it. Also, you can complement the monthly savings by investing a portion from bonuses. It works!

As the following table shows, at an 8 percent fixed annual rate of return, a family with a newborn baby that has approximately eighteen years of savings ahead of them will need to save approximately $3,500 every year (in today's dollars) for eighteen years to accumulate enough money to fund $15,000 per year (inflating at 5.1 percent) of their child's college educational expenses. If you start later, you'll need to save more annually.

Annual Contribution Needed, in Today's Dollars, for College Costs of $15,000 per Year for 4 Yrs. of College Funding Assuming a Fixed Rate of Return of 8 percent		
Current Age	Years to Save	Savings Amount
Newborn	18	$3,488.00
Age 5	13	$4,739.00
Age 10	8	$7,468.00
Age 15	3	$19,081.00

THOUGHTS ON RETIREMENT

We began this chapter overhearing two physicians in their seventies talking about their assets and wondering when they could retire from practice. Neither had saved enough in their pension plans to provide the kind of living to which they had become accustomed. Both of them certainly would have to sell assets and make radical changes in lifestyle in order to live on the income from a pension plan worth $150,000. That would produce about $6,000 per year at 4 percent and their social security payments would add about $20,000. Their ability to give to their favorite ministries would be markedly restricted and their ability to serve the Lord might well be unaffordable.

It behooves even the youngest practitioner to begin to prepare and plan for retirement as early as possible, to set some goals and indicators of progress along the way and to plan to spend his or her retirement years in activities that are productive for the kingdom of God.

Those who have planned carefully find that a retirement age of fifty-five to sixty years will leave at least ten years in which to serve God and the poor either overseas or in a domestic missions opportunity. Many who have so planned testify enthusiastically of the fulfillment and joy they experience using their profession as a means of expressing God's love to the less fortunate at home and abroad. Most of these serve as self-supporting missionaries.

The successful practitioner does not need to continue earning money that he or she could never spend, money that might be squandered by heirs. How much better to set a goal for a second career in ministry and spend the last years of practice exploring long and short-term opportunities for mis-

Those who have planned carefully find that a retirement age of fifty-five to sixty years will leave at least ten years in which to serve God and the poor either overseas or in a domestic missions opportunity.

Some doctors prefer to think of the time of retirement as a time of restructuring. God is always working in our lives and though we may cease our lifelong occupation, we will never cease to fit into God's plan as long as we are able to serve.

sions service or service to an organization that is proclaiming the gospel of Christ to those who will be eternally lost without it.

One CMDA member planned to retire at the age of fifty-five, having set that goal ten years beforehand. As his net worth increased and his giving increased, he completed the education of his children and retired at age fifty-six. Then he and his wife were led by God to serve on the foreign mission field and were financially free to do so. They learned a new language and a new culture. They were fascinated and blessed by the experience that, incidentally, invigorated their marriage.

Their first three years as self-supporting missionaries were funded by his partnership corporate stock buyout. For the next three years he took distributions—first, from his pension plan at fifty-nine and a half years of age, and then from social security at age sixty-two.

These two retirees were accepted as full members of the missionary family on that field and took on the serendipitous roles of surrogate grandparents for missionary children and counselors to missionaries suffering from discouragement and burnout. Upon leaving the mission field, the doctor was led by God to a position with a mission organization, where he has served without salary over the past ten years.

Some doctors prefer to think of the time of retirement as a time of restructuring. God is always working in our lives and though we may cease our lifelong occupation, we will never cease to fit into God's plan as long as we are able to serve. Here are some worthwhile thoughts on the restructuring of our lives under God's guidance:

- You will never retire from God's service—be ready financially to serve
- Be prudent, but trust God with your heirs
- Curb consumption; find ways to reduce spending and simplify your lifestyle
- Give more after your kids are educated; trust God with your financial security
- Set your retirement age based on God's plan for your life, not on your work fatigue and financial security
- Become debt-free
- Plan the future of God's money through estate planning.

When your entire life is offered up in God's service, retirement is just a change in venue.

PLANNING YOUR ESTATE

The Stewardship Ministry of CMDA is always looking for information and resources that can be used to equip or encourage our members and friends to be the best stewards possible. Recently a study stated that seven out of ten Americans did not have an estate plan and seven of ten with a will were not satisfied with their current plan.

How can this be? For many it's because they claim they are too busy with life, they feel like they have too little property, that it's expensive, or that they don't like dealing with attorneys or legal documents. While no one enjoys talking about death, all of us are mortal and sooner or later we are all going to die.

As followers of Christ, we should keep in mind that this whole idea of wealth and accumulation is not about us, but about our ability to be good stewards over that which has been entrusted to us. In many ways, our lives are like a tapestry woven with many choices—what occupation to pursue, where to go to school, who to marry, and how to worship. Though we have the freedom to make choices, many fail to make some of the most important ones out of apathy or procrastination. Estate planning is a good example of this.

Estate planning is up to each individual. We have the opportunity to make critical choices, which include saving taxes, minimizing administrative costs, preserving assets, and, most importantly, how our spouse and children will be cared for. Most of us feel we would do a better job at making these decisions than Uncle Sam would, yet by not taking the time to plan, we leave many of our privileged decisions up to someone else.

The Stewardship staff of CMDA has had the privilege of visiting with many families in different stages of planning their estates. Conversations often center on the question of how much is enough to meet their needs and to leave for their children and grandchildren. The next generation has the potential to become the wealthiest in a family's history. This is partly due to the growing financial markets and moreso because of the preceding generation's understanding of the value of money. Sadly enough, the next generation could also become the poorest through the consumption philosophy this world is placing in their hearts and minds.

In working with families to develop strategies for their estates we have seen parents wrestle more with the issue of providing an inheritance than any other single issue. These struggles often arise because tradition tells us that to provide a good inheritance we should pass on as much as possible to future generations. Sometimes we simply desire to provide something for our children that we did not enjoy.

Recently a study stated that seven out of ten Americans did not have an estate plan and seven of ten with a will were not satisfied with their current plan.

In today's economy, the equivalence of a biblical inheritance would be providing an education and the ability to earn a living.

When we examine the Scriptures, many passages speak about this issue. The most direct passages were penned by the apostle Paul. He wrote, "If anyone does not provide for his relatives, and especially for his immediate family, he has denied the faith and is worse than an unbeliever" (1 Tim. 5:8). So what is one to provide? In addition to a spiritual legacy, Paul is probably referring to those basic needs of food, shelter, healthcare, and a good work ethic. He also wrote, "If a man will not work, he shall not eat" (2 Thess. 3:10). From these passages we learn there is a balance to be maintained between giving our children what they need and making them dependent on what we give.

In today's economy, the equivalence of a biblical inheritance would be providing an education and the ability to earn a living. For some of our children, leaving an inheritance larger than the amount necessary to get them started with a good education will diminish the drive and energy they might need to become independent stewards of God's blessings in their lives. Be certain you have prayerfully considered your children's needs within God's plan for their life of service as you plan your estate.

Besides planning our estate for our children's benefit, one of the many privileges we have as Americans is the opportunity to give to charity what we would otherwise have to pay to our government in estate taxes. Most of us would probably prefer that an effective ministry spend our money after we are gone rather than the government. Our laws allow us this option. For this reason the CMDA Stewardship Ministry offers to help doctors with tax-wise strategies for income tax and estate planning. Our responsibility to use our money wisely for God's kingdom does not end when we escape this world for heaven.

A CMDA member attended an estate and planned giving seminar sponsored by the Stewardship Ministry. At this seminar the CMDA member was introduced to several planning strategies designed to give to kingdom purposes what might otherwise be paid in income tax, capital gains tax, or estate taxes. Finding the need to sell a parcel of highly appreciated property, this member decided to look at these options. This resulted in a plan that will allow his family to sell the property and give over $750,000 to advance the kingdom instead of benefiting Washington. Now that will bring real joy!

Another family was surprised to learn that under their current estate plan they would pay in excess of three million dollars in estate taxes. "How can this be, and why has my current financial advisor not helped me plan better?" was this mature doctor's immediate response. Over the next four months the Stewardship Ministry provided educational materials and assisted this medical couple in choosing a professional advisor who helped them implement a plan resulting in lowering the amount they currently pay in income tax, avoiding thousands of dollars in capital gains tax, and moving 100 percent of the three million dollars to kingdom purposes.

When asked if they were comfortable with the proposed plan, including a significant gift to charity, the doctor's reply was, "That's what I have worked for all my life. Why would I not be comfortable with advancing the kingdom?"

Remember that we live our lives within an eternal time frame—with the redemption of the world as our chief purpose in life. We must not limit God's use of our financial resources to our few decades of life in this world or to the benefit of the small cluster of people that we call family. We must trust God with our family and with the power of our money for his purposes, even after we have gone.

Here's a checklist that might be helpful in summing up the message of this chapter.

*Adopt a thoroughly Christian worldview
*Regard money as a means to an end, not an end in itself
*Develop and adhere to a financial control plan
*Tithe and give according to your covenant with God
*Take advantage of the incentives for long-term savings and let compounding work for you.
*Educate yourself in financial principles that will allow you to gain ownership of your situation
*Seek professional counsel on financial matters from a counselor who is both honest and competent
*Do not regard money and its accumulation as a measure of your self-worth
*Do not purchase by impulse and violate your financial control plan
*Do not make major purchases without multiple estimates and a cooling-off period
*Do not invest in ventures that both you and your spouse do not understand thoroughly and mutually support
*Do not buy and sell automobiles to assume an appearance of prosperity
*Do not neglect adoption of a careful estate plan before you enjoy heaven

Remember that we live our lives within an eternal time frame—with the redemption of the world as our chief purpose in life.

THREE QUESTIONS TO ASK YOURSELF
1. Who owns all of my money?
2. Who holds my security in his hands?
3. Do I know where all of my income goes each month?

THREE ACTIONS TO CONSIDER
1. Develop a mission statement for your money. Write down the bottom-line purposes for your income.
2. Prayerfully develop a plan that will enable your family to be out of debt by the time you reach fifty. Include education loans and your home mortgage in the plan.
3. Plan and modify your lifestyle so that within five years you will be able to regularly allocate over 10 percent of your income (before taxes) towards God's work in caring for the poor and in evangelism. Ask God if this is his will for your family, and then do it if he says, "Yes."

PRAYER

Dear Father,
I don't know why you have given me this life and all within it. Thank you. Thank you. Thank you. Make me faithful. Make me content. Make me wise. Make me responsible. Let me pour out my life for you as you have poured yours out for me. Let me never forget your cross or my home in heaven.
                                                                            —Amen

CHAPTER 12

The Hurting Doctor

He worked beside us for years – pleasant, competent, a doctor like all others we knew. We used to chat with him in the doctor's lounge, and we occasionally saw him on the tennis court or at church. His patients loved him. One day we realized we hadn't seen him lately. Someone said his house was for sale. Patients that we shared with him told us that he had taken a leave of absence from his practice and his partners were following them until he returned.

One day he was there again. He looked unchanged, except his wedding ring was gone, and he didn't joke so much. He never talks about his time away.

Doctors bend and break just like all other human beings. They lose their families, become depressed, develop anger, and drug addiction just like other people. Somehow we don't expect it, and then it happens to us or to one we know. It even happens to Christian doctors. We and our communities hold up an imaginary image of doctors that confuses us when we see a doctor hurting.

Dr. Roland Gray with the Physician's Health Program of the Tennessee Medical Foundation outlines the following myths that often make doctors legends in their own minds:

- Physicians should be all-knowing
- Uncertainty is a sign of weakness
- Patients should always come first
- Technical excellence will provide satisfaction
- Physicians are immune to illness
- To reveal emotions is a weakness
- Physicians don't have needs

*"Don't
let
your
'Pudgy'
die."*

Some doctors believe these and other similar myths. But, within the legendary land of these myths, the doctor exists as a real person, pounded by a real life with extraordinary pressures, leading to huge levels of personal stress.

Dr. David Allen, a Christian psychiatrist, relates a Bahamian folktale that pictures the plight of the hurting doctor:

THE PARABLE OF PUDGY

Pudgy was a little fish that lived on the western end of Nassau in the Bahamas. His parents warned him that he shouldn't swim too close to the shore because the large waves, especially around the month of October, would kick him up onto the beach and he would die.

But Pudgy knew best. As far as he was concerned he could swim better than his parents or siblings. After all, he had gone to a better swimming school than all of them. So, against the advice of his elders, one October morning Pudgy went swimming close to the beaches on the western end of Nassau. A large wave tossed him up on the sand, and as he watched the water ebb away, he realized he was beached. He flipped his tail. He twisted his body. He tried to jump off the beach, but try as he might he was unable to get back into the beautiful aquamarine sea. Afraid and trapped, he now remembered all his parents had told him.

As the Bahamian sun grew hotter, water evaporated from Pudgy and he became weaker. As the morning wore on, Pudgy went into early shock. He tried and tried to get back into the water but the waves lapped just short of him, leaving him stranded. His heart beat faster and his fear now turned to terror.

Along the beach came a very sophisticated lady. Fascinated by the spectacle of the little fish on the beach she stooped down to tell him how excited she was to meet him. But even before she could open her mouth Pudgy blurted out his plea for help, "Please help me, I'm beached. Put me back into the water – a fish out of water will die."

"Oh," said the lady, "I understand, but you see I belong to the Bahamas Independent Society and we believe that if people are just given the chance to help themselves they can handle their problems much more effectively. In fact, I am on my way to the Independent Society meeting at our church down the street. So little fish, you just keep on trying and I'm sure you will be able to do it all by yourself."

"Please help me," said Pudgy. "You don't even have to love me; just kick me back into the sea."

"Don't be preposterous," said the lady. "I would never kick one of God's little creatures. In fact, I volunteer at the animal society weekly. God knows I would never harm a vulnerable little animal like you, so don't think like that. Just keep

on trying. You know the saying, 'Try and try again, boys, and you will succeed at last.' Anyway, I must be off to my meeting now – but I'll stop by on my way back and we can discuss your position further. Cheerio, and have a good day."

Pudgy tried again and again but became weaker until he could hardly move. Then Pudgy died, and when the tide rose that afternoon, it took Pudgy out to sea.

A little later our lady returned to the beach to check on Pudgy. When she arrived at the spot where Pudgy had been she exclaimed in a loud, joyous voice, "I knew he could do it, I will never forget that little fish. He is now swimming with all the other little fishes in the Bahamian sea. He had a problem, and just like we said in our meeting this morning, he faced it. Now he is swimming happily ever after with all the other fishes in the Bahamian sea."

But Pudgy was dead.

Pudgy can be a wife who calls and warns us that she is hurting, but because we are so busy we don't hear her. Pudgy can be a husband who is hurting, but because we are so busy we don't hear him. Sadly, Pudgy can also be our children, who under much pressure at school and play, cry out to us sometimes by negative behaviors like drug abuse or even delinquency. But most of all, Pudgy can be our own heart that warns us time after time to take care of a certain problem, to get help for a certain addiction, to get more help for the office, to slow down, or to spend more time with our spouse or our children. But so busy, we turn a deaf ear and our heart hardens, and Pudgy dies.

When some students in the first-year at Georgetown Medical School heard this parable, they coined the motto, "Don't let your 'Pudgy' die."

In the early part of medical school, our heart is open and very innocent. We are ready to learn and be caring and see the patient as a person. But somehow, as the years go by, our heart hardens, our Pudgy dies and we lose contact with ourselves and our family and sometimes even our patients. And for some, the story of Pudgy becomes the story of their hearts.

CAUSES OF OUR PAIN

Dr. Allen has identified a number of common issues that seem to be common sources of pain in the lives of doctors in modern medical practice:

1. Litigious Environment. A litigious environment is a major concern for many doctors in many parts of the world, but particularly in America. Medicine, though rapidly moving to become a science, is still very much an art. It is too easy for even a good doctor to make a mistake that results in a

In the early part of medical school, our heart is open and very innocent. We are ready to learn and be caring and see the patient as a person. But somehow, as the years go by, our heart hardens, our Pudgy dies and we lose contact with ourselves and our family and sometimes even our patients.

It is possible for doctors to try their best to do the good and everything not turn out okay.

malpractice suit. I often find doctors of strong Christian convictions who pass through the process of malpractice and are left with a "tale of hurt" involving anger, bitterness, and disgust. Sometimes such anger is deflected onto their families, their practices, and certainly their personal lives. The doctor becomes somewhat defensive instead of being creative in the practice of medicine.

I remember vividly a very good doctor who suffered through a malpractice suit brought against him by a certain lady. He remembers testifying in court and remembers hearing his patient testify, and, even though he won the case, he said his heart burned with anger toward her. He became depressed; he couldn't sleep; he began isolating himself from his family and church. He had a dream one night and in the dream he literally watched someone he assumed was a surgeon cut open his chest; his heart bled profusely while the surgeon was trying to stop the bleeding. His fear was that the surgeon would fail, and the person would die. On awakening, he understood that the malpractice experience had left a bleeding wound in his heart. He realized that his non-forgiving attitude toward the patient was causing his heart to continue to bleed; he realized that if he did not let go the pain of not forgiving, that pain would eventually destroy him. He told me that in his prayer life he came to a place where he had to forgive her in order to let the pain go. What struck me was the sincerity and the pain I observed as this doctor related his story.

–David Allen, M.D.

It has often been taught in medical school—do the good and everything will be okay. It is possible for doctors to try their best to do the good and everything not turn out okay.

2. Depression: Many doctors have come to me with clinical depression. It comes on suddenly; sometimes it happens earlier in practice, but most often it occurs throughout the forties and fifties and is associated with the pressure of the work and the pressure of the family. In some cases, the doctor may have a bipolar depression that has lain dormant for many years; then something occurs in the practice like a financial loss, the death of a particular person, a malpractice suit, or the loss of particular staff, and that event precipitates the bipolar episode.

I've known doctors to become depressed because of an action they couldn't live with—an affair with a staff member or a wrong decision with a patient. As a result, their home life was wrecked and they committed suicide.

We doctors are human and we do get depressed. It is important for us not to self-medicate but to seek help to get the depression treated. Depression tends to be recurrent and relapsing. I have worked with doctors who have been through multiple episodes of depression that have left them bitter and angry toward life.

3. Addictions: For more than twenty-five years I have worked in the field of cocaine addiction. It is amazing how many doctors suffer from various types of addictions. The most common substances range from cocaine to Percodan; of course Oxycodone is very, very popular. The doctor tends to be very competent. Generally speaking, there is a problem at home and he or she seeks refuge in this particular drug. Many doctors have strong egos, so it is really hard for us to admit that we have a problem.

One particular doctor developed a narcotic problem, and after I spent four days pleading with him to get help, he said, "I would like to get help, but I am building my practice. I have a lot of expenses, and if I take time off to get help, I will be thrown far behind." Notice the irrational, illogical thinking that occurs. In a case like this, forced intervention techniques must be used, however painful they are for the doctor, his family, and others.

Addiction may declare itself when doctors overwork and become very tired. For example, one doctor who worked very hard decided he would buy some Bristol Cream Sherry to help. He was not really an alcohol drinker but parked by the road and virtually drank the whole bottle to drown the pain and sorrows of his day. As he was driving home, he was driving dangerously, so was arrested and had to face a D.U.I. charge. For this doctor who lived his life as a perfectionist, this was a tremendous personal tragedy.

4. Boundary Issues: Doctors become tired, have issues with their family, and then it is not uncommon for boundary issues to arise. It may not get to the point where a doctor abuses a patient, but he/she may become over friendly towards a patient and give them certain privileges such as hiring them in the office. As an unplanned result of that, things get out of hand. This can be a very painful experience. Often underlying the action is some type of depression, exhaustion, or loneliness. One should involve others when working with the opposite sex; it provides consensual validation, which is very protective and helpful.

5. Marital Failure: Doctors work extremely hard and this puts much pressure on their wives/husbands and families. From my experience, doctors have a high rate of divorce or marital difficulties. Many times we doctors come home tired and our spouse wants us to share the happenings of the

The doctor tends to be very competent. Generally speaking, there is a problem at home and he or she seeks refuge in this particular drug. Many doctors have strong egos, so it is really hard for us to admit that we have a problem.

Doctors may become extremely defensive when being asked questions by their spouse instead of really leveling. One is usually defensive because one is trying to avoid lying while reconstructing reality.

day with them, but we clam up. Our spouses are surprised that we can open up to colleagues and be very kind to patients but be very distant and isolated with them. This puts tremendous pressure on a marriage and it comes out in many different forms.

For example, a doctor may be very critical: "You always cook poorly," he might say. Using the word "always" nearly always destroys the soul of the relationship. A doctor may show contempt by calling the spouse by a particular name, "You are a stupid person," or "You are fat." This contemptuousness has a way of breaking up the inner connections of relationship.

Doctors may become extremely defensive when being asked questions by their spouse instead of really leveling. One is usually defensive because one is trying to avoid lying while reconstructing reality. Finally, stonewalling occurs where some doctors just go silent and don't speak. One doctor explained to me that sometimes when he and his wife became angry he might not speak to her for two weeks at a time.

6. Problems with Children: Doctors are extremely busy. Children need stability, consistency, and predictability in order for them to bond and to grow into meaningful family members and to become good citizens. Many times we are so busy we just do not have the time to give to our children.

I will never forget the death of a very well-known colleague. He was deeply committed to his work. While making a night call to a patient at home he had a heart attack and died. A few weeks later his daughter consulted me. I was very sad because I loved her father; he was such a distinguished man. "I am so sorry to hear about your dad's death because he was such a great man," I said. And then she replied, "Dr. Allen, I know it is sad that my dad died. But the truth, is I never knew my father as my daddy, I only knew him as 'the great doctor.' He was everybody's friend. He was good for all his patients, but he never had time for me. I never knew him. He is gone and I want to miss him, but I am missing the missing of him."
—David Allen, M.D.

This kind of separation from our children suddenly happens and we have to check ourselves. Children certainly need money and they need lovely vacations, but more than anything else, we need to recognize that they need us. The sons are particularly difficult. Unless we spend time with our sons, they rebel. It has been shown through various research that it takes the father-son relationship to develop control issues that relate to addictive behavior, career choices, and sexual orientation. It is clear that one of the great lacks of a doctor in medicine is that sometimes we male doctors do not express love to our boy children.

I will never forget a presentation at a missions conference when a mother was describing how she covered up for her doctor husband who had apparently achieved greatness by doing many wonderful surgeries in a particular area of a foreign country. The mother said she would try to cover up for his lack of time with his children by taking the children to see him during the day. She felt that because she had taken that aggressive approach to making sure the kids saw their dad at work, somehow she had averted the tragedy of her kids missing their father. While she was telling this story, her son, now a lawyer aged thirty-five, jumped up in the meeting and said, "Mum, that is a lie! It is not true. You did not replace my father. My father hurt me; he was never there for me, and nothing you did replaced that. I was hurt then, I am hurt now, and there will always be a hole in my heart when I think of what I have missed in not having the closeness of my father." The whole audience went into tears over the inner void that was left because of this man's father hunger.

—David Allen, M.D.

...so with the frustrations, the anger, the decreased IQ, and now the loss of inhibitions from the alcohol, many times tragedies result involving domestic violence, impaired decision making, and other destructive behaviors.

6. Anger: Doctors face many frustrations dealing with their personal lives, their family and marital issues, their patients, difficult illnesses with complications, the particular atmosphere of malpractice, all complicated by the pressure of insurance and business issues so that this frustration or hurt produces a sense of anger. The anger is internalized and may lead to depression or it may just lead to a cynical view toward life.

Some doctors go into a rage when they return home because of the frustrations awaiting them there. This rage powers a physiological arousal involving a rise in blood pressure, and an increase in pulse rate, which is associated with a decrease in IQ. In fact, as the pulse rate increases about ten percent above normal it is possible for one's IQ to go down anywhere from twenty-five to thirty points. At that point the doctors may become irrational, leading to poor judgment.

Complicating the situation is that sometimes when doctors are very angry, particularly at home, they take a drink of alcohol and the alcohol reduces the inhibitions—and so with the frustrations, the anger, the decreased IQ, and now the loss of inhibitions from the alcohol, many times tragedies result involving domestic violence, impaired decision making, and other destructive behaviors.

Shattered dreams may also play a part. As doctors, particularly early in life, we have many expectations for ourselves and we think that by a certain age we should have achieved a certain status in one arena or another. When we realize that this has not happened, our dream shatters and we become angry and very frustrated. Internalized anger is a very painful thing; the doctor feels miserable, and becomes irritable and difficult to live with at

As doctors, particularly early in life, we have many expectations for ourselves and we think that by a certain age we should have achieved a certain status in one arena or another. When we realize that this has not happened, our dream shatters and we become angry and very frustrated.

home. All of this produces a painful, negative atmosphere in the home, which creates a vicious cycle of hurt.

7. Poor Business Decisions: Many doctors are not good business persons. Without the help of very good professionals, sometimes we make irrational or poor business choices which have painful consequences, e.g., sometimes a bankruptcy, the loss of a practice, or just having to live with tremendous debt. This pressure produces very painful effects in the doctor's life with a hurt that is very hard. Other doctors seem to be doing well in business and we feel somewhat jealous and the hurt is accentuated and becomes more and more painful.

8. Invincible Attitude: This is true for some doctors, particularly when it comes to their own health. They self-medicate, self-treat, and sometimes cause themselves great difficulty. When they do become ill, it is hard for many doctors to accept treatment.

When I was an intern, a famous doctor was admitted to the hospital with a heart attack. This doctor had helped many people and had become a hero for helping the poor. During his first night in the hospital, he tired of lying in bed, and to my surprise, he put on his clothes, shaved, put on cologne, and went out on the town. That night he dropped dead of a heart attack. He had helped so many people, but he had an invincible attitude toward his own health. He refused to obey the regulations his doctors had prescribed for him, so his sense of invincibility led to his demise.

–David Allen, M.D.

We can sometimes become very arrogant and with an illusion of invincibility find ourselves hurting much more than necessary because we fail to take the proper advice.

9. Retirement: Medicine is a very competitive profession and doctors are given deep respect and high status by society. Therefore, when a doctor retires, it is natural to miss the status and respect. Some doctors are very much affected by this and, upon retiring, feel displaced, lost, and not sure how to live in retirement. Many times a doctor does not plan for this and it seems to come on him very, very suddenly.

A major factor may be the spouse who is upset because the doctor is hanging around the house more than before. They are accustomed to being apart and the change requires a new kind of adaptation to being with each other.

It seems reasonable that doctors should not just stop working without looking for something to transfer some of their talent to in order not to suffer the pain of retirement.

False Intimacy: In addition to the issues above, the editors would like to add one more, which is a growing concern in society at large—false intimacy via pornography and other means.

Ours is a country where over ten billion dollars is spent by consumers annually on pornography, and some of those consumers are Christian doctors. Over two thousand five hundred new pornographic sites appear on the Internet every week. This is not free speech but obscenity that invades homes and wrecks lives, even the lives of the most faithful. Thirty-seven percent of pastors admit that they struggle with cyber porn.[1] Nine out of ten children between the ages of eight and sixteen have viewed pornography on the Internet, often unintentionally when researching for homework.

Pornography is addictive and holds onto its victims with a hold like that of a narcotic. Doctors are not immune. Like any other comfort measure, pornography may especially take hold of the lonely, tired, or hurting doctor. In doing so, pornography does not just soothe an imaginary need, it becomes a snake that poisons family and patient relationships; it becomes a new and terrible chain that enslaves a doctor, whom God created to help free the world.

SOLUTIONS

The pain of hurting doctors is both real and common. However, there are things we can do to protect ourselves and heal the wounds that have been suffered:[2]

♦Learn to relax and meditate
♦Practice acceptance
♦Make a gratitude list
♦Watch the use of alcohol and drugs
♦Talk to friends – develop a support network
♦Physical exercise
♦Maintain balance in life
♦Develop a positive attitude – see life as a challenge and an opportunity to grow
♦Open yourself to new experiences – try new things, food and places
♦Work on personal and family relationships
♦Take time off

Ours is a country where over ten billion dollars is spent by consumers annually on pornography, and some of those consumers are Christian doctors.

Our vocation as doctors is to open our hearts to the vision of God's love in the world.

•Develop hobbies – life outside of medicine
•Seek professional help when needed
•Personal accountability by a group or respected individual for areas of personal weakness.
•A reliable Internet filter (e.g., www.bsafehome.com).

THE ULTIMATE HEALING

In addition to taking the steps above, Dr. Allen sees healing coming through adherence to the following seven principles from the Last Supper:

1. Love – Jesus told his disciples, "I have loved you to the uttermost." The doctor may prescribe, the surgeon may operate, and the psychiatrist may listen, but only God's love heals. No matter how hurt we are…regardless of how we are feeling, we are loved unconditionally by God. This means we have meaning, dignity, value, and identity. Sadly many of us fear love because in the past, where we expected love, we received hurt. So now we may fear love because it may bring pain.

We are spiritual beings made in the image of God. God surrounds and sustains us by his grace and love. Our heart pain can be healed when we realize his love by opening ourselves to its vision and personally committing to follow the mission of God's love in the world. The vision without the mission is an empty hallucination. And the mission without the vision leads to busyness and burnout. Our vocation as doctors is to open our hearts to the vision of God's love in the world. Many times our career (mission) blocks our vocation. Getting our vocation and career in the right perspective makes a difference in our life and leads to the healing of our hearts.

2. Communion – At the Last Supper the disciples were engaged in communion. Communion is the basis for community and communication. So often we doctors suffer alone. Pain is hard, but when shared it becomes a little easier.

Communion with persons (derived from the Latin word "per" = through and "sonare" = to sound) allows us to benefit from the love, truth, and beauty that God is sounding through them.

Communion with God creates interior silence and provides space for an inward table set for God and ourselves, e.g., David could say "Thou preparest a table before me in the presence of mine enemies…" (Ps. 23:5, KJV). Communion with God moves us beyond *chronos* time (daily time) into *kairos* time (God's time). Commitment to God through kairos time removes the opaqueness of life and opens into the transparency of God's love. "The heavens declare the glory of God" (Ps. 19:1).

3. Resistance – When we are hurt, the world's resistance towards us becomes evident. Our awareness of that resistance makes us angry, frustrated, depressed, and sad. We need to open ourselves to these feelings, so they may have less of a hold on us. Remember that even as Judas was betraying Christ, God's work continued in spite of him. Let us likewise realize that God's work in our lives continues in spite of whatever resistance or problems we are facing. Let us not make idols of our failures or mistakes, but in God's name journey on – knowing that our labor in the Lord is not in vain.

4. Humility – At a certain point in the supper Christ humbled himself by taking off his outer garment. Humility is the healing grace. The word humility, derived from the Latin word *humus* (soil), means learning to accept ourselves as we are. It means being grounded in ourselves and God, the ground and source of all being. Scripture indicates that God is always closer when we become aware of our sin or failure. Sadly, humility is a very difficult experience for many doctors to achieve. The strenuous training of medicine, the respect given to us by the public, and the power of presiding over the illness of fellow human beings can give us what some have called a god-like complex.

The hubris of the doctor is a very important component of the character that drives us to achieve. Unfortunately, many times it is this pride that prevents us from receiving the healing that is already ours in Christ. Humility means coming to the point of giving up our pride, giving up our illusion of invincibility, and opening ourselves to the naked love of God's healing. It takes humility to admit that one has problems. It takes humility to seek help. It takes humility to continue in help and it takes humility to follow up on help. Without this sense of humility it is very difficult for the hurting doctor to receive the support that he or she needs. All life involves change, all change involves loss, and all loss involves pain. Whenever we allow the dynamics of change, loss, and pain to increase our pride, then our heart becomes hardened, making healing difficult.

Humility is essentially facing our life as it is, facing our problems as they are, facing our situation as it is. As we accept the truth of life as it is, God's love and grace come to bring healing. Humility opens us up to realize that we are limited and that we all are dependent on God's providence. Without humility our problems may become a god who is so great that the problems become unsolvable. But once we learn through humility to bow our problems before God, God then accepts control and puts our problems in the right perspective. Many times doctors hurt not because of the problem

The hubris of the doctor is a very important component of the character that drives us to achieve. Unfortunately, many times it is this pride that prevents us from receiving the healing that is already ours in Christ.

*Do we
need to
have three
offices?
Do we
need to
have three
homes?
Do we
need to
hate the
lifestyle
we live?*

itself, but because somehow we have elevated our problems to god-like status, making healing impossible unless the only true God can overcome them. Humility means putting the problem in the right or proper perspective. "If God be for us, who can be against us?" (Rom. 8:31, KJV).

5. Simplicity – At the Last Supper, our Lord, after taking off his garments and demonstrating deep humility, takes a basin of water. It is so important for us as doctors with our tremendous technological training and the power invested in us to recognize that life, at its heart, is simple. In fact, life itself is grace; if we just hold our breath a few minutes, we won't be here. Forgetting the simplicity of the truly important aspects of life, we let the complexity of our work, the hustle and bustle of making and developing a practice, the business issues, complicate our life beyond our ability to comprehend or control.

Some years ago I worked with a very distinguished professor of medicine who was dying of cancer. Her word to me was this: In spite of the pathos and the pain, dying is very simple. There is no need for long talks or conversation or complex relationships or meetings. Unexpectedly, after being very ill, the professor was healed of the cancer and returned to health. She told me then that she wished she could live in health like she had lived when she was dying. "David," she said, "remember that life at its heart is very simple. When we are facing death only the basic things are necessary. Once we move out of illness we complicate our lifestyle and live beyond our means and make life more difficult for ourselves."

–David Allen, M.D.

Many doctors move around way too much. Do we need to have three offices? Do we need to have three homes? Do we need to hate the lifestyle we live? Have we tried to simplify our lives with a simple devotional period? At its heart, life is simple, and recognizing this helps us appreciate God's grace and love in a deeper way.

6. Service – Once our Lord had stripped himself of his outer garments and obtained a basin of water, he began to wash his disciples' feet. This is our finest picture of servanthood.

As Christian doctors, we see ourselves as servants, but when we hurt it is difficult to serve. We need to understand that even as our hurt immobilizes our service, Christ is still serving us—still washing our feet. He sends colleagues to encourage us, he sends us servants to bless us, he comes to us through our family, he comes to us even through difficult situations, even through failures in our practice, but he always comes because he came to serve.

Like him, even in our time of pain, we should seek to maintain our identity as servants. Serving others from within our pain is a commitment to follow the Christ who served others in his time of greatest pain. Our attitude, wherever we are in life, should be to serve each other, to help our brothers, to help our sisters. Many times we as doctors are very independent and so proud that we find it hard to ask other doctors to figuratively wash our feet. Some of us are so proud we find it difficult to wash the feet of other doctors. But it seems to me that our Lord was teaching us that when we wash the feet of those we serve, we in some sense also heal our own hearts. In other words, healing is a mutual process. As we care for others we find ourselves being cared for. As our Lord served his disciples so we, too, have to learn to serve each other.

We need to understand that even as our hurt immobilizes our service, Christ is still serving us—still washing our feet.

7. Transcendence – Our Lord told his disciples that he was leaving, but that after he left, he would send the Comforter. For the hurting doctor it is important to realize that God is still present, and therefore, there is hope. If we become our own god, we limit the resources that are available to us. Once we recognize that God is in charge, there are endless rays of hope. Transcendence means there is hope beyond our own ability and our own finite understanding.

Many times, we become so mired in our work, in our education, and the accolades of our profession, that we think we are "it," that everything begins and ends with us. And as a result, we forget that there is transcendence. There is a force greater than us. There is a God. There is a creator. When the hurting doctor becomes limited by his/her own perspective and ignores the presence of God, the pain becomes worse and the situation moves from hope to despair. It is so important to recognize that there is transcendence in the world. After we have tried to do everything that we can do and even when there is nothing else we can think of doing, God's love and grace still operate, bringing healing and hope.

Once upon a time a young boy visited a sculptor's studio in Rome. The boy noticed the sculptor chipping away at a huge marble block. To the little boy it seemed like a waste of time, and he wondered what the sculptor was doing. He asked the sculptor, "Why are you chipping away at the marble?"

The sculptor said, in a loving way, "Well, why don't you come back in about three weeks and see what I am doing." And so three weeks later the little boy went back to the sculptor's studio and to his surprise the block of marble had become a beautiful lion.

*If you are
hurting,
if you are
breaking
or have been
broken,
be wise; seek
help; seek
fellowship
and
accountability;
offer your
pain to God,
and ask for
his comfort
and guidance.*

The little boy in his surprise and shock said to the sculptor, "How did you know there was a lion in the marble?" The sculptor in a humble way said, "I knew there was a lion in the marble because before I saw the lion in the marble I saw the lion in my heart."

Before we can see the meaning of God in the world, we have to appreciate him in our hearts. As we open our hearts to God, Christ in us, the hope of glory, allows us to see God in the world. This connection completes the circle, and so regardless of how bad our situation is, or how difficult our pain may be, that circle of hope gives meaning and direction.

The chips of marble falling off the block as the sculptor worked correspond to the kind of pain we experience as believers and doctors. The chipping away of the marble by the master sculptor, God, is never easy. Sometimes it seems chaotic. Sometimes it seems as if it is going nowhere. Sometimes the suffering seems endless. Sometimes the pain seems hopeless. But as we wait, one day we will see the lion in the marble.

One day we will see that the God in our heart is the God in the world. The Bible says, "now we see through a glass, darkly, but then face to face..." (1 Cor. 13:12, KJV). We will come face to face with him, the true ground and source of our being, and in so doing, in a very deep sense, come face to face with ourselves.

In this light then, the sorrows and suffering of life give hope. As Paul wrote, "For I reckon that the sufferings of this present time are not worthy to be compared with the glory which shall be revealed in us. (Rom. 8:18, KJV).

If you are hurting, if you are breaking or have been broken, be wise; seek help; seek fellowship and accountability; offer your pain to God, and ask for his comfort and guidance.

THREE QUESTIONS TO ASK YOURSELF
1. What aspect of your life as a doctor causes you the most pain?
2. Refer back to Dr. Allen's teaching regarding the causes of our pain. How has your pain affected your life?
3. As God continues to chip away at the marble of your life, what greatness will he uncover?

THREE ACTIONS TO CONSIDER
1. Make a list of the forces that cause you the most pain in your personal and professional life.
2. Take your list to your pastor or spouse or a Christian colleague this week and pray with them for wisdom.

3. Recruit an accountability friend to help you overcome the hurt that keeps you from running the race God has laid out for you.

PRAYER

Dear Father of mercy and power,

I am in pain. I don't understand it all but I know you are here with me. Give me wisdom. Give me the strength to seek help and follow through. Be with me in power. Protect my family through it all. Help me come through this and rise stronger than ever before because I rise with you at my side.

In the name of him who was broken for me—Jesus.

—Amen

NOTES:

1. *Christianity Today*, Leadership Survey, December 2001.
2. Adapted from the work of Dr. Roland Gray.

CHAPTER 13

Malpractice

"...and fourth, that the doctor being himself a mortal human being, should be diligent and tender in relieving his suffering patients, inasmuch as he himself must one day be a like sufferer." –Thomas Sydenham (1624-1689)

A s the jury filed in, I thought: What could God possibly have in mind for this scene? Over and over the verse kept echoing: "You meant evil against me, but God meant [this] for good" (Gen. 50:20, NASB). Throughout my trial, the absurdity of my presence in the courtroom kept coming out. I had nothing to do with the missed diagnosis. I had referred Mary to three different ENT physicians for her smoking-related hoarseness, and all three had found nothing. When the diagnosis of metastatic laryngeal carcinoma was finally made, I was as surprised as anyone. Apparently the cancer had "hidden" just out of sight for over a year, but there it was. I had prayed with Mary before and after the diagnosis, for her marriage first and then later for her health.

Her husband had never been there for her during her illness, but after she died, disfigured by the radical surgery to remove the cancer, he had come to my office. Angry, guilty for his years of neglect, and very self-righteous, he knew who had killed "his Mary" —me and all my cronies. Try as I might to help him with his anger and frustration, nothing changed. The suit that followed was expected, but here I was, sitting in a courtroom eight years later, with two ENT surgeons, defending my honor before a jury of my peers.

Peers? I never will forget the first day of the trial. On the front row was a young man, maybe twenty-one years old, with a tee-shirt on that read "Armadillos Rule"...whatever that means. But at least he paid attention. The elderly lady on the back row had often just dozed. I felt as if my fate was truly in the hands of God, since the legal system seemed to have failed, at that moment, to give me the justice I deserved.

In fact, many reputable physicians of the era felt that medical liability cases would "weed out" incompetent physicians in a way that state and professional regulatory agencies had failed to do.

The decision was given to the judge and read: "No liability." Suddenly, I looked at the jury differently—they were smarter than I thought! In fact, as I found out later, Mr. Armadillo Rules was my biggest defender during the deliberations. I looked around the courtroom: My wife smiled wide enough to light up the room.

But no one cheered, no balloons were released, no confetti was thrown. We all filed out, said goodbye, and quietly promised ourselves never to speak of this again. Had I won anything after all? Where was my justice?

—Curt Harris, M.D.

ON THE ORIGINS AND HISTORY OF MODERN MALPRACTICE LIABILITY

In the United States, there have been five periods of history in which the number of medical liability cases filed increased rapidly;[1] the first was from 1840-1860. Early in the nineteenth century, general changes in the civil liability law (tort law) encouraged a nearly ten-fold increase in the number of medical malpractice cases filed. One of the most important changes was the approval by the courts of contingency fee arrangements. This opened the legal system to the poor, and was part of the turn-of-the-century egalitarian movement in the United States, influenced by the French Revolution.

Prior to this time, a patient injured by a physician's incompetence had to have the money to hire an attorney to represent him, and the patient would bear the entire cost if the case was lost. In practical terms, this excluded a large number of cases that could have been brought, simply because the injured patient was not wealthy. Since one of the founding principles of our nation was free access of all citizens to the courts, this change was widely applauded. In fact, many reputable physicians of the era felt that medical liability cases would "weed out" incompetent physicians in a way that state and professional regulatory agencies had failed to do.[2]

From the earliest moments of our current liability law, the two central goals of medical malpractice policy were: physician discipline through economic penalties; and provision of financial aid to help the patient injured by substandard care. Arguably, these goals have never been met well by our tort law, with each successive period of increasing liability somehow intended (at least in part) to address one inequity or another within the system. As an example, between 1890-1900, socially responsible physicians began to purchase a (then) new form of insurance, medical malpractice insurance, to both protect themselves against loss and to provide insurance money to their patients should they be injured by a mistake or substandard care. However, because this created more "wealth" subject to a finding of liability, malpractice law became a lucrative field of legal practice, and the number and types of malpractice cases soared. More injured patients received help, but the cost was borne entirely by the medical profession, forcing up the cost of medical care.

Without examining each period of "crisis," suffice it to say that each was strongly associated with improvements in the medical standard of care, with technological advances, and with increased complexity of therapy. These advances in medical practice occurred just as the general tort theories of legal liability expanded to include such concepts as joint and several liability, products liability, non-economic damage awards, and (later) informed consent.

Two major social changes during the last thirty years of the twentieth century are of particular importance to our current situation. There continues to be a growing distrust of all authority, a general questioning of the intentions and motivations of anyone with power over our personal autonomy. This emphasis on "me and mine" has been expressed in our public life by an acceptance of a secular system of values, based on individual freedom and morality, replacing the former Judeo-Christian system of values that are based on individual accountability and public virtue. These two changes have heightened our assignment of human blame for all things "wrong" in the world, and have lowered traditional barriers to using our legal system to solve our personal problems. If our laws and political beliefs do in fact reflect our personal and public values, we have changed.

In summary, each malpractice "crisis" in our history has not been associated with a worsening quality of medical knowledge or medical care, but rather with an improvement in medical practice. Arguably, the single most important determinant of the number of cases filed against physicians in each period was the development of standards of care against which physician behavior could be judged, and with improvements in the treatment of previously untreatable diseases. Both factors increased the risk that an individual physician could make an error in a complex treatment protocol that was subject to discovery and legal liability. Finally, the current emphasis in medical care on personal autonomy is part of a changed worldview that includes an increased demand for professional accountability, and a tacit assumption that any "bad outcome" is both unexpected and culpable. The burden of proving that a medical complication was not due to incompetent care has shifted to the physician—a heavy burden, indeed.

LAW, ACCOUNTABILITY, AND THE ART OF MEDICINE

Based on the brief discussion above, it has been the success of medicine as a profession (in an environment of increasing legal and social accountability) that has created what many physicians consider the "nightmare" of medical malpractice. By establishing standards of care, based on scientific

In summary, each malpractice "crisis" in our history has not been associated with a worsening quality of medical knowledge or medical care, but rather with an improvement in medical practice.

We understand how hard it can be to deal with the uncertainties of medical care, and we fear the worst while praying for the best. The dark secret we share is all we do not know and cannot do.

data and techniques, and by practicing medicine with the expectation of improving the health of our patients, we assumed responsibility for an outcome. As a profession, we talk about cures and treatments, sometimes as if we expect only the best. Today, medical practice is a mature discipline, and physicians consider themselves responsible for a high quality of care within that discipline. We understand how hard it can be to deal with the uncertainties of medical care, and we fear the worst while praying for the best. The dark secret we share is all we do not know and cannot do.[3] While recognizing the uncertainty of medical care and all of our profession's limitations, it is nonetheless our heart's desire to be judged fairly by others, and to be judged by our Creator as "good and faithful servants." The disappointment comes when we are judged unfairly by others. While this should come as no surprise, it is nonetheless painful when it happens.

Accountability for the patient's welfare has always been a central tenant of medical care, but unreasonable or random accountability is a too frequent part of our current legal system. Unwarranted cases are brought and won, based on legal trial tactics rather than true fault, while at the same time many instances of substandard care never draw attention. Anticipating which patient will sue for which problem continues to be unpredictable. Fear of the mere possibility of legal liability that is outside the physician's control builds an emotional barrier between the physician and his or her patient, a barrier that interferes with normal communication.

Unfortunately, preventing liability has become part of the art of medical practice. Physicians are taught to "talk to their patients" in order to avoid liability by improving rapport. Defensive medicine, generally defined as doing things not directly intended to benefit the patient but rather to avoid some perceived liability, is too common. Many state medical licensure boards require a formal knowledge of various liability issues in order to receive a license to practice medicine. Chart documentation is judged adequate more often by legal standards than by medical standards. Confidentiality of medical information is now defined by law rather than by professional standards of care or by patient needs. Legal liability issues were once "other than" the practice of medicine, but no more.

One problem caused by this incorporation of law into medical practice has been a new way of defining the moral equivalence between legal liability and medical error: If there is no legal liability then there is no medical error, and only those errors that result in legal liability "count."[4] When we hear of another physician who has been sued, we often assume it is something he or she deserved all along and is late in coming. We ignore our own mistakes as mere oversights, or imagine we are practicing error-free medicine. Only when one of our patients suffers greatly, or when we are sued, do we think about our day-to-day practices.

Most human errors are not preventable by redoubled personal efforts, and most medical errors do not breach any professional or moral standards. Therefore, we do not dwell on our errors because we do not look on them as a personal problem, nor do we value them highly enough. We only learn from those mistakes that have consequence. The Scottish poet Robert Burns once wrote "Oh that [God] would give us the gift to see ourselves as others see us." Is this the one gift that most of us would decline?

The Personal Side of Malpractice

I first met Mark during my residency in internal medicine. He was a young, aggressive and well trained emergency room physician practicing in a medium-sized rural town. He was married, had two young children, and had earned a respected place in his community by working nearly five years in the ER of the town's major private hospital. Mark painted in oils better than most commercial artists. I still have a small painting he gave me of two geese in flight hanging in my office.

One busy night, the town's popular sheriff came into the ER with burning chest pain. Mark examined him: his lab work was normal, but Mark missed a small "wiggle" on the EKG that suggested cardiac problems. By 3:00 a.m., after observation and testing, the sheriff was sent back to his squad car with a bottle of Maalox and reassurances. An hour later while on patrol, he crashed into a light pole, dead from a massive heart attack.

In the suit that followed, Mark was treated to the worst of the judicial system. He was publicly humiliated, cast in the light of an uncaring, grossly negligent and greedy physician. Abandoned by his social and church friends, unable to talk to anyone about how he felt, he began drinking. The eventual decision against him was for $2 million, twice his malpractice insurance.

His wife, in an effort to save her children, filed for divorce. On the day of the divorce hearing, rather than suffer another loss, Mark killed himself with his pistol. I am embarrassed to admit I only heard about Mark's death months afterward.
–Curt Harris, M.D.

Several studies have confirmed the effect of malpractice litigation on the individual physician. These include increased rates of depression, sexual dysfunction, divorce, drug and alcohol abuse, and suicide. These problems are well known. Less often understood, though, is the nearly uniform reaction of physicians to an iatrogenic bad outcome, whether or not a suit is

Most human errors are not preventable by redoubled personal efforts, and most medical errors do not breach any professional or moral standards. Therefore, we do not dwell on our errors because we do not look on them as a personal problem, nor do we value them highly enough.

"We see the horror of our mistakes, yet we are given no permission to deal with the enormous emotional impact; instead we are forced to continue the routine of repeatedly making decisions, any one of which could lead us back into the same pit."
--David Hilfiker, M.D.

brought, whether or not substandard care was involved. These include a sense of isolation from friends, deep remorse and grieving for the injured patient, anxiety, loss of self-esteem, and guilt (moral culpability). In 1984, David Hilfiker published an important, now classic article entitled "Facing Our Mistakes" in which he wrote: "We see the horror of our mistakes, yet we are given no permission to deal with the enormous emotional impact; instead we are forced to continue the routine of repeatedly making decisions, any one of which could lead us back into the same pit."[5] For the last eight years, CMDA has offered a counseling service for physicians facing malpractice litigation.[6] Our experience is that most physicians desperately need someone to talk to about how they are dealing with the situation, to shed the sense of isolation they feel. Although medical and legal literature have correctly described the common emotional responses to both malpractice and to iatrogenic complications, these problems are underestimated in both frequency and severity by most authors.

Our current malpractice "crisis" is fueled by the emotional brutality of the current tort system, which is based on an adversarial model of blame and shame. Our current approach is to ask "Who did what terrible thing wrong to whom?" in a world where simple errors are not only prevalent but are an intimate part of the human condition.[7]

THE NATURE OF HUMAN ERROR

It is neither possible nor necessary to review all of the theory and research on human error. Much of the information on medical error has been published by Dr. Lucian Leape,[8] and more recently by The Institute of Medicine. But a few simple statements are necessary.

First, we are not concerned here with intentional acts that cause an injury. Such acts are not mere negligent acts, but are criminal. Nor are we concerned with acts done with such a degree of disregard for possible harm that the acts could be called "gross negligence." Rather, we are concerned with ordinary negligence, or ordinary errors that lead to harm, without the intent of harm.

Broadly speaking, there are two kinds of activities we all engage in every day: skill-based activity and knowledge/rule-based activity. Skill-based activities are things we do that we have done many times before and are now very skilled in performing. A simple example is driving a car. Most of what we do when driving is based on long experience, including the route we travel. If we are unavoidably distracted from part of our driving, for example by a child suddenly crying in the car, and make an error, we have committed a skill-based error. But assume for a moment that somewhere on the route we have driven many times before, the signs on an intersection are changed from a four-way stop to a two-way stop. If we proceed through the intersection assuming an approaching car will stop and are hit by the other car, we have made an error and caused an injury during a rule-based activity. Skill-based errors occur most often in situations of distraction or fatigue; rule-based errors occur most often in situations of over-extension of our knowledge, or of not knowing what we do not know.

The greater the skill and expertise in any endeavor, the more we rely on skill-based activity (and less on rule-based activity); and the fewer errors we make. "Practice makes perfect." The more highly trained and experienced a physician, the less likely he or she is to make a "simple" mistake. However, this also implies that errors made by this same physician will occur in two common situations: (1) those he or she has not seen before and fails to recognize as unique, or (2) those in which the data necessary to respond correctly are unavailable, due to an unavoidable distraction or a failure in an information system.

Further, most human error (whether skill-based or rule-based) occurs due to "systems" problems (latent errors); that is, accidents waiting to happen. A common example of a series of latent errors was the sinking of the Titanic: There were inadequate lifeboats for the number of passengers, there was no shakedown cruise, the radio was inadequate to receive warnings of ice, and there were no "lids" on the watertight bulkheads to prevent overflow one to another. All of the skill-based or rule-based activities necessary to avoid the disaster were (arguably) performed at the moment the ship began to sink, but to no avail.

In medical practice, information is critical. When data are missing, misreported, or misinterpreted, error occurs. The reasons for each of these data problems are not infinite, and normally can be addressed . . . if the problem itself can be identified. But this is exactly where the current tort system is most damaging to any possible improvement in the quality of health care. If an error is always a "bad thing" and if individual blame must be assigned for the error, the possibility of change becomes remote. Until we view medical errors as valuable information, change will be unlikely or very slow, systems will not improve as rapidly as they might, and the focus will remain on improving individual performance by punitive measures. As a result, mistakes will not decrease.

THE ELEPHANT IN THE ROOM: FEAR OF LITIGATION

Much has been made of the real and significant cost of "defensive medicine." Physicians do perform tests they consider less important to avoid lit-

Until we view medical errors as valuable information, change will be unlikely or very slow, systems will not improve as rapidly as they might, and the focus will remain on improving individual performance by punitive measures. As a result, mistakes will not decrease.

There is often a fine line between tests that are not "cost-effective" and tests that are done under the banner of "defensive medicine." In fact, neither term is useful in a discussion of the quality of care a given physician provides, but they are political terms used by various groups to further their own goals.

igation, to be a little more certain of some diagnoses, or because certain tests represent a "traditional" standard of care. While such tests are an expense to a burdened healthcare system, there is nonetheless a value in such behavior: occasionally, a less probable diagnosis is made or an atypical disease is discovered.

We can certainly decide as a society that such infrequent benefits of "over-testing" are not cost-effective and thus limit the use of a test or procedure. But for the individual patient who is either reassured by a normal test or receives an early and unexpected diagnosis, the money was not wasted. There is often a fine line between tests that are not "cost-effective" and tests that are done under the banner of "defensive medicine." In fact, neither term is useful in a discussion of the quality of care a given physician provides, but they are political terms used by various groups to further their own goals.

However, even if we accept the idea that defensive medicine exists and excessive costs are caused by such behavior, the fear of litigation is far more damaging to the quality of medical care than mere dollars. Fear of litigation interferes with normal physician-patient communication, and therefore valuable information is lost. This both increases the probability of error, and decreases the probability that any error actually made will be critically examined for its cause. The cynical phrase "Doctors bury their mistakes" is true...as it applies to any open discussion of a medical error that might lead to litigation.

Fear of litigation also forces physicians to select the cases they will or will not treat, often leaving high-risk, ill patients without medical care. And fear of litigation, combined with the dollar cost of malpractice insurance that covers high-risk medical care, forces physicians to discontinue certain procedures or not to see certain patients. The undiscussed factor in certain care decisions is the fear that something will go wrong and the physician will be blamed. "Better just let nature take its course. You can't sue God."

Most physicians try hard to practice error-free medicine (or nearly so), and believe that, in the main, they achieve that goal. Therefore, they treat a mistake as unique, an aberration in an otherwise near-perfect system. In the face of a mistake, they promise themselves to redouble their efforts to attain perfection, but normally take no measures to correct any underlying cause of the mistake.

They sincerely believe the statement they make in the face of a bad outcome: "I did everything humanly possible" because it is normally true. But since perfection is impossible, errors recur. Fear of litigation drives normal corrective behavior underground.

THE PROBLEM OF PERFECTION IN A BROKEN LEGAL SYSTEM

Too often, it is the severity of the injury (the damages) not the nature of the error itself that determines if an error is "bad enough" to gain our attention. We focus on classes of errors rather than types of errors, and thus lose valuable information on how to avoid the same mistake over and over again, at some different time and place. The same mistake made in the care of a thirty-five-year-old mother-of-three as opposed to the less "sympathetic" seventy-five-year-old homeless woman will get a very different analysis. Human error is ubiquitous but not egalitarian.

Physicians correctly view malpractice litigation as a "lose-lose-lose" endeavor. The physician loses time, emotional energy, and money. The patient loses time, emotional energy, and money. The legal system loses dignity, respect, and authority. Lose-lose-lose. If the purpose of the tort system is to fairly compensate parties who suffer avoidable iatrogenic injury and to deter high risk or incompetent physician behavior, then the system usually fails.[9]

Many physicians (and others expert in medical error management) contend that: (1) most iatrogenic error goes undetected and uncompensated; (2) some litigation is baseless in terms of either standard practice or causation; (3) the current system is wasteful and unnecessarily expensive (only thirty to 40 percent of all dollars spent reach the injured patient); and, (4) litigation indirectly damages patient care by penalizing the most highly trained, procedure-oriented physician while at the same time ignoring the marginally competent (usually non-procedural) physician.

They point to the fact that several studies seem to say that the physician most likely to be sued is: well-trained, competent, in practice for more than five years (therefore at an increased risk due to the number of patients seen in that time), and somewhat less charismatic or personable–quite the opposite profile of the "bad apple" physician who seems to avoid litigation.

Malpractice insurance and litigation have become merely a "cost of doing business" unrelated to the quality of care delivered or to social equity. By ignoring the vast number of patients who deserve help, and by rewarding the clever and persistent patient and attorney, the legal system loses the moral force of any argument based on equity and justice. Can the system of justice be changed?

THE ROAR OF THE LION

In Africa, when hunting gazelles, the old, toothless lions crouch on one end of a field and roar, driving the game to the other side where the young lions quietly wait for the kill. From this comes the African saying: "Safety comes from running into the roar of the lion." It is hard to face our fears, to

Physicians correctly view malpractice litigation as a "lose-lose-lose" endeavor. The physician loses time, emotional energy, and money. The patient loses time, emotional energy, and money. The legal system loses dignity, respect, and authority.

The problem with such advice is that we are being told to manipulate our patients so that when we commit an error they will not sue us, because they like us, or that they will somehow feel personally responsible for the bad result since they participated in the decision making.

deal with difficult things when we should. But if we are to avoid being sued and survive a suit when we are sued, we must.

Avoiding the Suit

You have heard advice on how to avoid being sued: "Talk to your patients, tell them what they need to know, involve them in the decision, and build rapport." There is nothing wrong with that advice, as far as it goes. The problem with such advice is that we are being told to manipulate our patients so that when we commit an error they will not sue us because they like us, or that they will somehow feel personally responsible for the bad result since they participated in the decision making. Risk-management and error prevention share some goals, but not all. Your insurance company wants to keep the money you pay them. You want to avoid errors and lawsuits. The goals overlap but are not the same.

Please understand that the following suggestions are not risk management suggestions, but are biblical principles applied to our practices:

♦First, discipline your heart and mind, as Paul said in Phil. 4:8 "Finally, brothers, whatever is true, whatever is noble, whatever is right, whatever is pure, whatever is lovely, whatever is admirable–if anything is excellent or praiseworthy–think about such things."

♦Second, live by the two commandments of Christ, "Love the Lord your God with all your heart and with all your soul and with all your mind. This is the first and greatest commandment. And the second is like it: Love your neighbor (Ed. patient) as yourself" (Matt. 22:37-39).

♦Third, as the outworking of these two commands, examine your practice for quality and errors. Ask someone else to look at your practice and make suggestions as to how you can avoid errors, such as calling a wrong prescription or being in such a hurry that errors are easily made. Listen to your staff, and ask them to help you. Be transparent.

♦Fourth, imagine you are your patients, and ask what it feels like to be a patient of yours. Is the staff friendly? Do you keep people waiting only to rush through the appointment? Do your patients feel like they matter to you beyond getting past the appointment? Do you go the extra mile? Do you listen? Do you create an atmosphere of concern? Do you create a secure environment that encourages conversation? Do you pray for guidance to help them, and do you pray for their best?

•Fifth, don't structure your practice in a way that creates problems. Look at the system within which you practice. Build in redundancy and cross-checks at all decision-making points. Don't make financial arrangements that compromise the patient's welfare, such as contracts that require brief, technically-laden visits without personal contact, or pay you for withholding care.

•Sixth, if you make a mistake, and if you can make something right, admit the mistake and make the thing right. Often, it is the concealment of error that causes the patient to lose trust, to feel betrayed, and to sue you.

•Seventh, give patients a chance to honestly tell you how you are doing. Questionnaires are not a good substitute for a phone call to a patient who has left your practice angry. Make changes based on what you learn, rather than rationalizing away a complaint.

Think about what these ideas applied to your practice would mean. Better communication leads to fewer errors, leads to fewer bad results, leads to fewer lawsuits. You can't control everything. You may be sued nonetheless. But if you have studied how errors are made and how to avoid them, the simple advice just given you will ring true.

Scary? You bet it is. But not as frightening as sitting in a courtroom.

How to Survive (and thrive) During a Lawsuit

There is no substitute for spiritual maturity. Trouble brings spiritual maturity as nothing else can. As the old Baptist pastor once said: "When God brings you tribulation, he expects you to tribulate!" Shakespeare said it more eloquently: "He jests at scars who never felt a wound." The best gauge of our faith is the meaning we give to suffering. Will we be true to our faith, or deny it in order to avoid pain?

A Christian radiologist I know was sued for incorrectly reading an MRI. After several weeks of careful consideration and research into the accusation, he decided that he had made a mistake. An expert was then found by his attorney who was willing to testify that the error was nonetheless within the normal standard of care, and not malpractice. Again, he thought about it, and did research. He decided his attorney's expert was probably wrong. He went to his attorney and told him to settle the case, but his attorney refused. This time after careful prayer and thought, he again went to his attorney and told him that if he took the stand, he

If you make a mistake, and if you can make something right, admit the mistake and make the thing right. Often, it is the concealment of error that causes the patient to lose trust, to feel betrayed, and to sue you.

This doctor had done something he had never seen another doctor do in all his years as an attorney: Admit he was wrong. When he found out that it was because of the doctor's Christian faith, the attorney began to look at his own faith, and he realized something: He had not admitted his own wrong before God or his wife.

would become a witness for the injured patient—that Christ had commanded honesty and he could do no less. The certainty in the eyes of the physician and the reference to his faith forced the attorney to settle the case for the limits of the policy, one million dollars.

The physician, my friend, came to me two years after the suit settled. His insurance had gone up in price, and he had suffered some professional embarrassment from his public admission of responsibility. He wondered what the meaning of it all was: Why had God brought him this grief? He was not certain he was competent. He had begun to second guess himself all of the time. He wondered if medical practice was really what he should be doing. Maybe he should "retire to teaching."

I told him two things that changed his thinking and put a spring back into his step. First, I reminded him that only incompetent physicians feel they never make mistakes, and that he actually had a great reputation for being competent. But more importantly, I told him something he did not know, that I had heard a month before without making the connection to my friend. I had recently seen the attorney who had represented the patient in the suit against my friend. (I had known this attorney for years, and had not really respected him. He had said he was a Christian, but had behaved badly toward his family and wife.) When I saw him, I knew something had changed. He was back in his church, had rededicated his life to Christ, and had reconciled with his wife. I asked him what had happened. He told me about this Christian doctor he had sued, a radiologist, who could have hidden behind his expert and his lawyer, but had not. This doctor had done something he had never seen another doctor do in all his years as an attorney: Admit he was wrong. When he found out it was because of the doctor's Christian faith, the attorney began to look at his own faith, and he realized something: He had not admitted his own wrong before God or his wife. He was convicted by what my friend had done; he had seen real faith in action.

—Curt Harris, M.D.

It is important to remember that suffering may or may not be about us. It may be about how we represent Christ to others. We are not the center of the universe, nor are we the center of human suffering. Other, more important things may be happening.

Six principles for surviving and thriving during a malpractice suit:

•First, center everything you do on your faith. Don't pray for an easy life, pray to be a strong person. Pray as Christ did: "Abba, Father . . . everything is possible for you. Take this cup from me. Yet not what I will, but what you will" (Mark 14:36).

•Second, understand your emotions. It is common, even normal, to feel betrayed, isolated, angry, devastated, withdrawn, insecure, unappreciated, tired, and powerless. The "system" is out to get you. It is not paranoia when someone is really there. Don't blame others for the way you feel. Don't imagine that others know how you feel. Don't imagine that others are looking at you badly. The suit is not about your honor or dignity; it is about how you honor God.

•Third, don't expect fairness or logic from the courts. They are only as good as the flawed people who traffic in them. Trust in the Lord, pray for your attorney, and the patient and his/her attorney. Do not seek their demise. Pray that good will come of it all. Seek the prayers of others you trust. Lean on God.

•Fourth, if you made a mistake remember that everyone makes many mistakes, virtually every day. You have just been "found out" this time. Tell you attorney how you feel. Settle the case if at all possible. Remember that winning your case is not really a victory. Someone you cared about (your former patient) lost. There are no winners in malpractice suits, just judgments.

•Fifth, try to learn from the experience. Look at it as something of value, and find the value in it. It is there, if you are not blinded by hate or fear.

•Sixth, remember that you are a Christian who happens to be a doctor, not a doctor who happens to be a Christian. Take your responsibility to others seriously, but don't take yourself too seriously. Maybe a malpractice suit is a wake-up call that your reputation is not what is at stake, but that of our Lord. Self-assumed honor and dignity are illusions we make for ourselves, to give ourselves personal worth. Honor the Lord; rest on his grace and forgiveness.

CONCLUSION

The medical liability system is broken beyond simple repair. Major reform is needed and inevitable. While any reform must balance a patient's rights against the cost to the provider (and thus the cost of healthcare), the unaddressed issues of equity, fairness, and justice make most current proposals fatally flawed.

In all circumstances, a Christian physician must remember that medicine is a calling from God, and his or her first duty is to the patients who trust

Take your responsibility to others seriously, but don't take yourself too seriously. Maybe a malpractice suit is a wake-up call that your reputation is not what is at stake, but that of our Lord.

Our patients are not "the enemy." We must remember that we are all our own worst enemies, and do what is right and true, rather than compromise our faith.

their care to them. Our patients are not "the enemy." We must remember that we are all our own worst enemies, and do what is right and true, rather than compromise our faith. While being sued for malpractice is a painful situation, the opportunity for growth in our Christian life can be unsurpassed.

Christ taught us "all of the law" in two statements: "Love the Lord your God with all your heart and with all your soul and with all your mind. This is the first and greatest commandment. And the second is like it: Love your neighbor as yourself."[10] Do we really need more?

QUESTIONS TO IMPROVE CARE AND REDUCE YOUR CHANCE OF BEING SUED

1. What can I do to improve patient communications in my office? Specifically, what can I do to make certain that my patients, as they move through each step of their encounter with my office, feel that their problems have been heard and addressed?

Imagine your most difficult patient: How would a phone call or a visit go for him or her? As you imagine each step during a patient encounter in your office, consider one key question: Whose agenda is being served by this part of the encounter? If you identify any problems that concern a patient, quickly pray (either silently or with the patient) for the wisdom to deal with the issue well.

2. How can I be certain that I have addressed all of the problems that needed to be solved with each patient encounter?

There are issues your patient may not know about or care about that are important. Routine checklists based on standards of care can be very helpful here. Examples might include simple things like flu vaccinations and blood pressure checks, or complex issues like cardiac evaluations and referrals. These kinds of decisions should be as automatic as possible, leaving you with time to think about more important issues.

3. Finally, do I regularly meet the family members important to my patient, and ask them to help me with helping the patient?

This step is often overlooked, but can be the most important step to understanding who your patient really is, in his or her "real life," which is often different from the narrow impression he or she wants you to see. The more information you have, the less likely you are to make a mistake. Strongly encourage your patients to bring others with them on each visit. A refusal to do so may also give you an important clue about a dysfunctional home life.

ACTIONS TO TAKE WHEN THINGS GO WRONG

Pray for guidance and for God's words to be in your heart, in your mind, and on your lips. Throughout the process, lean on God. Then:

1. When one of your patients has an unexpected complication of his or her treatment or disease, as soon as possible, discuss with the patient and any and all family members what you know, but don't speculate about anything and don't try to blame another physician or caretaker. Be honest, be transparent, and be available, including after hours and off call. When you know more about what happened, and especially when you know more about what can be done to make things better, tell the patient and the family. Keep them informed as the care progresses.

2. If you are sued for malpractice, don't read the summons you receive beyond your name on the header. It will contain a lot of legally-required language that will make you angry and depressed, since most of the allegations in a summons have only a thin relationship to the truth. Inform your malpractice carrier; carefully secure and protect every scrap of paper relating to the care of the patient; and, print out a hard copy of any information stored on your computer, including billing and appointment information. Never, never, never add to or modify a record after you have been sued, since it will put every part of your records in question at trial. If you want to make notes separate from the chart, do so with your attorney, so what you do will be protected by the attorney-client privilege.

3. Talk to your spouse about how you feel; be completely honest—trust that your relationship will survive. (Your conversations will be protected from discovery later by the spousal privilege.) Too often, physicians (both men and women) feel that their spouse will think less of them if they made a mistake, and try to hide behind a series of half-truths. Silence can destroy a marriage.

If you are not married, talk to your pastor, a counselor, or someone close to you about how you feel. If you are talking to someone other than your spouse, avoid discussing anything but the public facts of the case, and focus on your emotions. These conversations will be of no value to the plaintiff's attorney, if he decides to discover them later.

4. Finally, a separate word or two for the spouse of a physician who has been sued.[11] Your spouse will be moody, angry, sometimes withdrawn, and occasionally inappropriately elated. He or she may feel that you cannot understand what is happening . . . and at one level, this is likely true, if you

> *Talk to your spouse about how you feel; be completely honest—trust that your relationship will survive.*

Look at the lawsuit as an opportunity to show your spouse how much you really love him or her—this is a moment of "worse" in the "for better or worse" part of your vows.

are not a physician or nurse—a person who has dedicated their life from an early age to being directly responsible for another's health. Therefore, it may be hard to understand the degree to which a malpractice suit threatens the very being of your loved one. However, you are the most important person in your spouse's world in every way.

Understand that it is very unlikely that you will lose your home, job, or position in the community because your husband or wife has been sued. If you start obsessing on that possibility, look at your own values, and ask yourself if you are living too much for "things." Keep your own mental and spiritual health sound, and get good counseling for yourself, if you need to.

Any problem you had in your marriage before the lawsuit was filed will probably be exaggerated, at least at first. Look at the lawsuit as an opportunity to show your spouse how much you really love him or her—this is a moment of "worse" in the "for better or worse" part of your vows.

Perhaps most importantly, realize that virtually every mood change, angry word, or insensitive act is not about you, but is about the malpractice suit and how it is hurting your spouse. One simple question can save a marriage: "Honey, are you upset with me or is it something else?"

5. If you need more help, call CMDA and ask for the Medical Malpractice Ministry. The number is 423-844-1000.

PRAYER

Dear God,
I don't understand why this is happening to me, but I know that you do. Teach me. Show me what you want me to do. Keep my heart and mind on you. Keep me from anger and bitterness. Protect my loved ones from anything I might say or anything that others might say that would hurt them. Forgive any wrong committed against me, and use it for your glory. In all of this, Thy will be done on earth as it is in heaven.

—Amen

NOTES:

1. The five periods of time recognized as associated with rapidly increasing numbers of cases filed are: 1840-1860, 1890-1900, 1920-1930, 1960-1970, and 1975-1985. See James C. Mohr, "American Medical Malpractice Litigation in Historical Perspective" *Journal of the American Medical Association* (JAMA) 283:1731 (April 5, 2000). Many authorities believe we are currently experiencing the sixth period of increasing liability, and date the beginning of this "crisis" as

2001. For a recent discussion of the impact of law on medical practice, see Sara Rosenbaum, J.D., *JAMA* 289:1546 (March 26, 2003).

2. In 1850, William Wood, M.D., US Navy officer and physician, complained that the increase in malpractice claims against well-trained physicians instead of self-proclaimed practitioners was misdirected. (Alternative medicine practitioners and, in some measure, incompetent physicians seemed to avoid all liability.) "It is better to be without a diploma . . . to be able to say, 'I make no pretensions, I only gave my neighbor in his suffering what aid I could.'" By establishing standards of care and by practicing according to those standards, reputable physicians made themselves targets for claims of malpractice. Alternative care practitioners (e.g. homeopathic medicine, herbalists, and health food advocates) typically do not claim to cure or treat any conditions, but rather to merely "help in some way," leaving the ill to judge by the standard of "let the buyer beware" the quality of the help they have received. However, Congress is considering increasing the power of the FDA to regulate such practices through its licensure and approval processes.

3. The nineteenth century cynic and humorist Mark Twain hit at the heart of this secret when he wrote, "God heals and the doctor takes the fee." For a more sober reflection, see "Facing Our Mistakes" David Hilfiker, M.D., *New England Journal of Medicine (NEJM)* 310:118 (January 12, 1984).

4. Part of this assumption is based on a defensive, adaptive response to the personal emotional pain a physician suffers when one of his or her patients becomes ill or dies despite all best efforts otherwise. To assume the responsibility for every "bad outcome" is simply too painful for most, if not all, physicians, so an emotional screening process to avoid doing so necessarily occurs. For a classic study on the effect of perceived errors on physicians' emotional health, see John Christensen, Wendy Levinson, and Patrick Dunn "The Heart of Darkness" *Journal of General Internal Medicine* 7:424 (July/August 1992) (examines the emotional cost of medical errors and iatrogenic bad outcomes even in the absence of liability or fault).

5. Hilfiker, op cit.

6. The name of the service is the Medical Malpractice Ministry of the Christian Medical and Dental Associations (CMDA). For more details, contact CMDA at their national offices in Bristol, Tennessee (423) 844-1000.

7. Christian physicians feel all of the same emotions as do non-Christian physicians, with this added: Since we approach our medical practice as a service to our Lord, we have a "double" sense of failure. First, we blame ourselves for the errors we commit, based on hindsight. "If only I had been more careful there, or done that here." Additionally, we feel that we have somehow failed in our dedication to Christ through our profession by making an error. The problem is this: We can always find something wrong with ourselves for those unintended mistakes we make every day. But it is arrogant to even imagine that we can be perfect in anything. The realization that we are imperfect sinners, prone to error, is the beginning of humility. And the beginning of wisdom is true humility (Proverbs 11:2).

8. Lucian Leape, M.D. "Error in Medicine" *JAMA* 272:1851 (Dec. 21, 1994).

9. For a strong argument that the current legal system is "broken" see Philip K. Howard "Is the Medical Justice System Broken?" *Journal of Obstetrics & Gynecology*

102:446 (Sept. 2003). See also Michelle M. Mello and Troyen A. Brennan, "Deterrence of Medical Errors: Theory and Evidence for Malpractice Reform" *Texas L. Rev.* 80:1595 (2002); Frederick Levy, M.D. "Tort Reform: 'Evidence', Politics and Policy" *Legal Medicine Perspectives* 12:53 July/Aug. 2003; also see Barry R. Furrow, et al. *Health Law* (4th ed) 2003 Supplement, pages 80-85. When reading the various publications on this debate, you may be reminded of the quote by Andre Lang: "He uses statistics as a drunken man uses lampposts . . . for support rather than illumination."

10. Matt. 22:37-40. As Francis Schaeffer has written, love is truly the "mark of the Christian."

11. To my knowledge, the topic of how a malpractice suit affects children has not been studied. However, it is probably safe to note that the attitude of the parents toward the suit, and how they allow the suit to effect their marriage, is critical. Children take their lead from their parents, and will usually feel the need to defend a parent accused of a wrong. Be certain to talk to your children about what is happening: otherwise, they may believe that they somehow did something to cause all of the anger and frustration they see. Reassure them about their safety and security, and how much they are loved.

CHAPTER 14

Marriage and Family

R *on and I recently celebrated our twenty-fifth wedding anniversary. I am a pediatrician and Ron has worked in budgets and finance for that computer company that kept getting bought – Digital, Compaq, and now HP. Ron finally took the retirement package and called it quits. Our two girls are off to college and graduate school, so you would think that we would be at a great place in our married life. Marriage is great, but we still struggle with priorities, personality differences, communication, sex, romance, and keeping God in the center of it all. You'd think we would have figured it out by now. We have made progress over the past twelve years, once we realized our marriage had been going in the wrong direction. We've seen the "big D" word happen to too many of our friends and my patients' families. We decided not to let it happen to us.*

—Patti Francis, M.D.

Marriage takes a lot of work. But it is important work and God must think that it's important work since he uses marriage as an example or a metaphor so often in the Bible. From Genesis to Revelation, it is clear that marriage was his idea—after all, we see in Genesis that he created Eve to be Adam's mate, and in Revelation believers are invited to the wedding supper of the Lamb, symbolizing the ultimate union of Christ with his beloved—the church.

In between these texts, God's original marital intent and the final marital blessing, lies the state of marriage in our world today – broken and wounded due to the sin of our human nature. Yet God pursues us with unconditional love. Marriage stands as a mirror to the world of this grace of God. Two sinners are wed together in marital blindness, and begin to see their selfish natures emerge. Life then gets a bit tough with overwork, sleepless nights, huge loans, in-laws, and children. In a God-centered marriage, con-

Marriage is one context within which God chisels away at our selfish idols and replaces each offering with himself.

fession, forgiveness, and grace become daily activities that lead to renewed intimacy with God and each other. God's grace is relived daily in the lives of God-centered husbands and wives.

Marriage is one context within which God chisels away at our selfish idols and replaces each offering with himself. Marriage can become a refiner's fire where we realize how much God can heal us of our brokenness. And as he heals us, he so often fills us with his presence and with the blessings that come from sharing a life with each other. That's God's work. But he also expects us to do our part.

How to Have a Great Marriage

◆Make marriage your priority

If you play golf, you understand that in order to improve your game, you need to give it time and attention. You need to practice your drives and your putts. It's the same with marriage. When you are engaged, you spend hours together and never run out of things to talk about.

By comparison, how much time do you spend as a couple now? Do you have a date night? Do you dream together? How do you share your faith together as a couple? We are all over busy and our world has an unending supply of distractions to occupy our time. Where in our order of priorities does our marriage fit?

Jesus identified the great commandment in Matt. 22:37-40: "'Love the Lord your God with all your heart and with all your soul and with all your mind.' This is the first and greatest commandment. And the second is like it: 'Love your neighbor as yourself.' All the Law and the Prophets hang on these two commandments."

In relation to marriage, our question might be similar to the one asked of Jesus after he made those statements: "If I am to love my neighbor, does that include my spouse?" Does love include time? Does love include focus?

Often the people we are closest to get the leftovers because we think they'll understand. So we see extra patients, teach medical students, attend committee meetings, serve on the elder board, go on mission trips. These are all good and important activities. But they are not more important than the one who is at home, waiting for us. Ask God to show you what you need to let go of and what you need to grasp with all your might. Find out where God has given you passion and gifts and go only to the things he has called you to outside the home.

To the rest of the stuff you should learn to say "No!" Be preemptive. Decide on your calendar how much time you should schedule with your spouse each week, and commit. You don't have to make excuses to anyone about this. Just like the phone message that says, "We can't come to the phone right now" you can say "I'm sorry, I'm not available then." Only you can be that husband or wife. There is no way around it; priority is spelled T-I-M-E.

John and Carrie lived in a rural town where Carrie home-schooled two of their three small children. One weekend they came to our marriage enrichment retreat with a common concern. John was in a busy family practice group and spent little time at home to help with the kids and participate in their education. Carrie felt burdened and alone with too much responsibility at home. As a part of our retreat we held an exercise and discussion about love languages. John was surprised to learn that Carrie's love language was "quality time." He realized that he didn't have any such time to give her, let alone to help out at home. They had to make a choice.

A few months later we received a note from John. After our retreat they had worked through several good discussions with prayer together about the future of their marriage and their family. John realized how important it was to Carrie that he be a partner in raising their three children. They sought the Lord's help, willing to change. God presented them with an opportunity to move to a different part of the country where John's work schedule would give him more time at home. It was a turning point in their relationship. Together they decided that their marriage and family were more important than John's job and they did something about it. John and Carrie were excited to see what God had in store for them.

–Patti Francis, M.D.

•Celebrate Your Differences

Another important aspect of enjoying marriage to its fullest is understanding your spouse's personality type and yours! You've heard "opposites attract," but once you're married, they can repel like bug spray! Be honest. Certain things you initially loved about your spouse really bug you now. But step back and take another look. Understand that people of different personalities see life differently.

There are many personality tests out there but we enjoy the one Gary Smalley has worked out in his book *The Two Sides of Love*. Most people have a primary and secondary personality profile and these will fall into four general types. Gary Smalley uses animals, presenting great word pictures anyone can understand.

Lions are dominant types, confident and decisive, good at getting things done. They are very result oriented. Stubbornness and big egos are their

Decide on your calendar how much time you should schedule with your spouse each week, and commit. You don't have to make excuses to anyone about this.

Another important aspect of enjoying marriage to its fullest is understanding your spouse's personality type and yours! You've heard "opposites attract," but once you're married, they can repel like bug spray!

weaknesses. Status and power meet their needs; they fear losing control and looking bad. They struggle with trusting God and letting him control things. Lions are good leaders and you always need one in any group setting to help get things decided and accomplished. The apostle Paul probably was a lion, as are many doctors.

Beavers are analytical perfectionists who are very logical and precise. Beavers will make sure you do it right! They are the ones who are most organized. But they can have trouble overanalyzing situations and struggle with decision making. To admit they are wrong is beyond comprehension! Failure destroys them. Grace is something they need to experience and hand out more freely. If you want order out of chaos, give the problem to a beaver.

Otters are optimists and motivators– the planners and life of the party! Their conversation is articulate and gregarious. They can be very emotional and reactive. Sometimes they talk a bit too much and worry about acceptance and recognition. Rejection destroys them. Being too impulsive can interfere with their waiting on God. But if you want motivation and some fun, an otter can make it happen! The biblical characters Peter and Barnabas were otters.

Golden Retrievers are what every friend wants. They are loyal, steady, sensitive, and patient. Compliance makes them easy and agreeable. Job security and stability is important. Change is disastrous. Conflict sends them running or withdrawing. They aim to please and are always seeking others' approval even though God's approval is a better place to invest their energies. If you want to keep the peace and have a loyal fan, marry a golden retriever.

Physicians and dentists tend to be lions or beavers. They need these strengths to get through school and residency! But they tend to marry otters or golden retrievers. The positive sides of such blends can be greatly complement each other. But when their excesses or struggles surface, watch out! A lion can be too dominant with a golden retriever who retreats or an otter can be too impulsive for the perfectionistic, hard-to-commit beaver.

When Ron (the beaver) plans our vacation trips, he researches absolutely every possible option of where to stay, so as to not make a mistake in his choice. It makes for a great vacation, but the process of his being on the computer for days on end,

and my having to look at each choice with him, when I (a lion) want to just make a decision, can lead to conflict (next section). It helps me to remember that Ron needs to go through this process; I can then appreciate him for all the time and effort he puts into it and recognize how much that side of him adds to our family.
—Patti Francis, M.D.

◆Learn to Handle Conflict Constructively

A couple's communication process often reflects the state of their marriage. In marriage enrichment weekends, working on communication is the most valuable session for most couples because it is the nitty-gritty of daily life. A physician or dentist usually has been communicating all day long and may come home disinterested in finding out about everyone else's day. A spouse at home with kids may be desperate for adult conversation. The result is conversation mismatch and conflict is triggered.

Bad patterns of conflict lead to unhappiness and distancing, which in turn lead to getting your needs met elsewhere – at work, in an affair, in community involvement, in the kids. All these substitutes destroy the intimacy designed for the marriage relationship.

In *Fighting for Your Marriage*, Markman, Stanley, and Blumberg described four key patterns of communication that can harm a relationship and lead to divorce:

1. **Escalation** occurs when a couple respond negatively back and forth, raising their voices and using increasingly more extreme comments as time goes on. If this pattern can be recognized in time, when one partner starts to escalate, the other person might soften their voice, back off on the negative and remain open to listening. This may lead the aggressor to de-escalate as well.

2. **Invalidation** is a pattern in which one partner subtly or directly devalues the thoughts, feelings, or character of the other. This hammers away at their partner's self-esteem. Our spouse deserves better treatment than that. It's always important to show your partner respect and listen completely to their point of view.

3. **Withdrawal and avoidance** are different manifestations of the same pattern in which one partner shows an unwillingness to start or stay with important discussions. If a spouse feels that withdrawal is necessary, they should state what they are feeling and why, before they leave. If needed, a time should be scheduled when it feels safer to talk over the issue.

A physician or dentist usually has been communicating all day long and may come home disinterested in finding out about everyone else's day. A spouse at home with kids may be desperate for adult conversation.

In order to turn poor communication into good communication one needs good listening skills, and must learn how to adequately express feelings and desires.

4. The final poor pattern of communication is **negative interpretations**, when one partner consistently believes that the motives of the other are more negative than is really the case. If you feel that your partner is always acting negatively towards you, don't assume that the intentions are negative; ask for clarification. Was it intended as negative comment or was there misreading going on? Most of such comments between loved ones are misunderstood and we each need to look for the positive comments as well.

These patterns of communication erode all good things in any relationship. In order to learn to communicate in more healthy patterns, you first need to identify the negative styles you each use. Try to understand how you each got there to begin with. Were they patterns that were modeled to you growing up? Were unmet needs driving you to frustration and therefore poor communication skills? Eliminate all "You…" statements and instead say "I feel this when…." This avoids all the blaming.

Prov. 25:11 says "A word aptly spoken is like apples of gold in settings of silver." And Prov. 18:13 adds "He who answers before listening – that is his folly and his shame." Finally Prov. 15:1 says "A gentle answer turns away wrath, but a harsh word stirs up anger." If you have significant anger issues, get help from a friend, pastor, or counselor. These feelings will alienate your spouse and destroy your marriage.

In order to turn poor communication into good communication one needs good listening skills, and must learn how to adequately express feelings and desires. When one of you initiates a conversation that needs some discussion, set aside the time to sit down together and really go through it. If emotions are high, postpone it until feelings are calm. The "Speaker – Listener Technique" is a good way to start.

Here's how it works. Let the initiator or speaker "have the floor" and state the issue. He or she should begin with:

1. "What I observe…" (facts on the issue),
2. "What I think…" (intellectual analysis),
3. "What I feel…" (emotional input), and
4. "What I want…" (expressing desires).

Next, the speaker may make a proposal with a plan of action. It is critical to conclude with the speaker assuring their partner of their commitment to the relationship.

The listener needs to maintain eye contact throughout and not interrupt with a reaction to any of their partner's comments. The listener then should reflect back to their partner what they heard with the speaker clarifying anything that was misunderstood. Then they trade places and go through the same exercise.

This has been a very successful process in marriage enrichment weekends. You can actually put squares on the floor with the above quotes and each participant couple can "walk" through an issue. This technique has proven helpful in solving such dilemmas as finding a parking place, getting to church on time, not missing an airplane flight, and buying a summer home or a dog.

There may be a time when a couple needs help in communication beyond books or exercises and that's when a good Christian counselor and a lot of prayer are needed. Years of bad habits don't resolve overnight, but such patterns can slowly change into a much healthier way to communicate. To do it well requires self-sacrifice and forgiveness that only Christ can supply.

◆Nurture Romance and Intimacy

In the typical couple, romance and intimacy to a woman mean dinner out with good conversation, and to a man they mean skipping the conversation and getting on to making love. When you think about love in marriage, romance and intimacy are the only parts of our lives that are exclusive to the marital relationship according to God's design. Yet they are the hardest to talk about on our weekend enrichment seminars! The Bible has some great romance and intimacy scenes throughout, starting in the Garden of Eden. The Song of Solomon has beautiful references to courtship and making love.

God made sex for us to enjoy, but somehow we get hung up after the kids start arriving and work gets demanding. So how do we get sex back to where it was on our wedding day? Learn how to spell R-O-M-A-N-C-E:

Revise your schedule. Get out your palm pilot and schedule time with your spouse. If it's not on your schedule, it won't happen!

Oneness in our relationship. In Steve Arterburn's book *Every Woman's Desire* he challenges men to understand what their wife's "essence" is; what are her gifts, thoughts, needs? Men, ask your wives what oneness means to her and then do it. It will make the next point really exciting!

Making love. If your sex life is in a rut, or making love is non-existent, then it's time to talk about it. Often, diminished sexual fulfillment in marriage is a symptom of other problems in the relationship. Or, there may have been some past abuse issue that has built a wall. Sometimes we are just carried away with our hectic lifestyle and making love gets left out in the

Years of bad habits don't resolve overnight, but such patterns can slowly change into a much healthier way to communicate. To do it well requires self-sacrifice and forgiveness that only Christ can supply.

When you think about love in marriage, romance and intimacy are the only parts of our lives that are exclusive to the marital relationship according to God's design.

cold. It's okay to schedule sex into your calendar if other priorities have crowded it out and you are too exhausted to be spontaneous.

Activities. Make dates, plan things you both enjoying doing together, or take up an interest that your partner enjoys. You can spend time exercising together or reading a book together. Refuse to let arguments spoil this time.

Needs. What are your spouse's top two or three emotional needs? In *Give and Take*, Willard Harley Jr. says that the top five needs of women are affection, conversation, honesty and openness, financial support, and family commitment. The top five needs of men are sexual fulfillment, recreational companionship, attractive spouse, domestic support, and admiration.

Conversation and **C**aring. Harley also describes how "love busters" destroy romantic love. These are selfish demands, disrespectful judgments, angry outbursts, dishonesty, annoying habits, and independent behavior. A beautiful romantic night leading to great sex can get sideswiped to separate bedrooms with any of these actions. In caring, learn your spouse's love language by reading Gary Chapman's book *The Five Love Languages*. There are five basic ways we each speak and understand emotional love. When someone we care about loves us in our love language, our emotional tank is filled and intimacy occurs. The love languages are: words of affirmation, quality time, receiving gifts, acts of service, and physical touch. Know your spouse's one or two love languages and then show her or him love in these ways!

Express & **E**xperience forgiveness. If there is no acknowledgment of sin and failure, and asking and receiving forgiveness, a marriage is guaranteed to fail. Paul reminds us in Eph. 4:32, "Be kind and compassionate to one another, forgiving each other, just as in Christ God forgave you." Col. 3:13-14 says, "Bear with each other and forgive whatever grievances you may have against one another. Forgive as the Lord forgave you. And over all these virtues put on love, which binds them all together in perfect unity." Learn to ask for forgiveness and learn to forgive.

You won't be able to work on all of these areas at once, but pick one that you both want to work on, read one of the recommended books and schedule some time to go over it. It will be the best gift you can give your marriage and your spouse!

✦Recommit to Each Other and to God

God has a great design for marriage that started in the Garden of Eden. He made us in his image, each gender reflecting and complementing his glory. He designed husband and wife to be co-laborers and intimate allies and to have a ministry to our broken, sinful world. But because of our own sinfulness and selfishness, we often give up in the struggle. It's just too much work!

God has persevered with us and calls us to persevere with each other. As we are obedient to that call, God takes our muddled messes and turns them into miracles, like diamonds of radiant beauty. This is a life-long process that takes time and is often painful. Heb. 10:36 says, "You need to persevere so that when you have done the will of God, you will receive what he has promised." Heb. 12:1-2, says "...let us throw off everything that hinders and the sin that so easily entangles, and let us run with perseverance the race marked out for us. Let us fix our eyes on Jesus, the author and perfecter of our faith...."

God wants to make our faith perfect, which in the original language meant "finished" or "complete." Most of us are a long way from that. The first step in moving the incomplete toward the complete is to recognize the flaws. Marriage is the perfect opportunity to discover our flaws (which our partner often points out to us freely!).

Once our flaws are discovered, we can admit them and ask for forgiveness. As we discover the freedom this process gives us in our marriage, we discover more and more one of God's great plans for marriage, that is, to develop within us the same truth, grace, and forgiveness toward a broken and chaotic world around us.

As we discover how to honor our spouse, build them up as a "Christ-bearer," and encourage their spiritual giftedness, we show the world how God's kingdom is meant to be. God's kingdom is portrayed to the world in a marriage where two broken and forgiving people stay committed to one another in a sacrificial relationship in the face of life's chaos.

In addition to living in this relationship of grace, we also need to pray for and with each other on a daily basis. Very few couples pray together, probably less than four percent. Why? Pride, insecurity, busyness, and distance are often the reasons. Yet when a couple prays together daily, the chance of divorce is less than one in fifteen hundred! Who wouldn't want that guarantee?

You won't be able to work on all of these areas at once, but pick one that you both want to work on, read one of the recommended books and schedule some time to go over it.

YOU CAN WORK ON THIS TOGETHER

So what are you going to do for your marriage? How are you going to love your spouse with a Christ-like unconditional love? How can you make God the center of your marriage? Take each topic above and decide individually and then together the short term (in the next few weeks and months) and long term (in the next months to years) goals you are willing to establish together.

God has persevered with us and calls us to persevere with each other. As we are obedient to that call, God takes our muddled messes and turns them into miracles, like diamonds of radiant beauty.

Answer for yourself, and together, the following questions:

♦What priorities are you willing to establish to enhance your marriage?
♦What areas of communication do you need to work on?
♦How can you spice up your romance and sex life?
♦How can you grow spiritually?
♦What does it mean to you to center your marriage on your relationship with the Lord?

If it's too difficult to talk about these things together, then seek help with a Christian counselor and marriage retreat weekend. (See the CMDA website: *www.cmdahome.org*.) Every time a marriage fails, God sheds tears. When our marriages fail, we miss his great plan. We miss the great blessings he has in store for us. For those who have experienced the pain of divorce, remember that God still loves you. The scare may remain, but God can restore purpose and joy to your life.

HOW TO BUILD GOOD FAMILY RELATIONSHIPS

My dad was a family practice physician and my younger brother is one. So I've been surrounded by medicine since the beginning. Growing up, I could see that my dad was married more to his work than to my mom, but she was faithful and accepted her role. I admired her for that over the years. When I was in college, I spent time in my dad's office. I learned about a whole other side to him! At home he had not been available emotionally and had rarely made it to any of my Scouting events like the other dads. But then I saw him with his patients; he was so caring and compassionate; they adored him. I realized that he had given his all to them and didn't have much left for us at home. Watching him at work helped me let go of my disappointments in him as a dad. Our relationship improved when I understood him better.

But I committed myself to being different, to being there for my kids in the future, even though I felt called to medicine. In my fourth year of medical school I became pregnant unexpectedly and this jolted me into prioritizing the family issue right from the beginning. I knew that God would make me a better doctor and mom by forcing me to make decisions early regarding the raising of my family. I would never regret the path God took us down even though it wasn't the one Ron and I had mapped out. (Kids were supposed to start in about year seven of our marriage!)

I wanted to be a mom first; so I've been fortunate to be able to work part-time. Obviously, my two girls would have had more of me if I was home full-time, but

I was confident that I had pursued God's direction after Corrie was born at the end of medical school. I very clearly felt God leading me back to part-time residency and private practice. Life has felt like a whirlwind of busyness from Corrie's first cry until our first year as "empty nesters".

Now it's much easier to sit back and reflect on the things we did right and where we could have improved. We did all we knew to do. We had read several books on parenting, taken classes, and said a lot of prayers (sometimes with tears).

There are no guarantees as to how any of our kids will turn out. The world pulls hard to separate them from us and from our Lord; but purposeful parenting will definitely make a difference, even if it takes years to see the fruit.

–Patti Francis, M.D.

In addition to living in this relationship of grace, we also need to pray for and with each other on a daily basis.

Guidance Parents Can Best Provide

As parents we are responsible to guide the development of our children in five major areas: **spiritual**, **relational**, **physical**, **emotional**, and **educational**.

♦SPIRITUAL DEVELOPMENT

Spiritually, we desire that our children know Jesus Christ as their personal Savior; that they be obedient to his call; and, that they live a life of holiness with love and compassion for God and others. You can sum these up in the Great Commandment in Matt. 22:37-40: "'Love the Lord your God with all your heart and with all your soul and with all your mind.' This is the first and greatest commandment. And the second is like it: 'Love your neighbor as yourself.' All the Law and the Prophets hang on these two commandments," and the Great Commission in Matt. 28:19-20: "Therefore go and make disciples of all nations, baptizing them in the name of the Father and of the Son and of the Holy Spirit, and teaching them to obey everything I have commanded you...."

We want our children's faith to be their own, so here are some things you might do in order to facilitate this:

- *Make Sunday God's day*. Even when they whine about it, take them to church. Make Sundays entirely a holy day from the beginning so as to establish that early on.
- *Read a children's Bible or stories about the Bible* when they are young.
- *Listen to "Adventures in Odyssey" tapes* (from Focus on the Family) on any driving vacation when they are younger. This is radio theatre with a Christian message and a Bible verse at the end.

There are no guarantees as to how any of our kids will turn out. The world pulls hard to separate them from us and from our Lord; but purposeful parenting will definitely make a difference, even if it takes years to see the fruit.

• **Pray for them often** as a couple and at the dinner table. Ask your kids how you can pray for them.
• **Work as a family** in a soup kitchen or with an inner city mission.
• **Help out with any mission trip** your church plans where one of your kids or your entire family can participate.

I was asked to participate as the team doctor (always in great demand) on our church's yearly Mexico trips when my girls were in high school. I've also taken one of my daughters on a Samaritan's Purse medical mission trip.
—Patti Francis, M.D.

• **Sign them up for Christian camp** every summer as early as they can go.
• **Model spiritual leadership**.
• **Conduct family devotions** on a regular basis (there's lots of fun material available to help with this).

Remember, you have the biggest influence on your children's faith. Make it a high priority to attend to the spiritual growth of each of your children. It's the best gift you can give them and the one with the best long-term return!

◆**RELATIONSHIPS**

We all want our kids to be happy with who they are and how they connect with others. Most of the brokenness in the world today, outside of not knowing the Lord, is the broken down state of family and friends. Think of all the people you know who are hurting. It is often because they don't feel loved or because they are suffocating from anger over being hurt. It is critical that we pay attention to the way our kids relate to us and to others. Here are some suggestions:

• **Love your spouse.** The best gift you can give your kids besides faith in Christ is a healthy marital relationship. When a marriage is solid and the husband and wife treat each other with respect and show love for each other, their kids feel secure and loved also. Most well-adjusted kids come from families with strong marriages. So work on your marriage!

• **Model forgiveness.** In your asking and receiving forgiveness, your children will see their own sinfulness and seek God's forgiveness ("…forgive us our debts as we also have forgiven our debtors" Matt. 6:12). They need to see that when we make mistakes toward them and our spouses we know how to apologize humbly, once we've admitted we're wrong.

• **Spend time with your children's friends.** As you do this over the years, you gain a sense of how they are choosing them. As the saying goes, "Show me your friends, and I'll tell you who you are."

We've occasionally had great discussions about what makes a good friend, especially after a friendship disappointment. This brings in the whole discussion of character education, which you must not neglect. Respect for others and their property, truth telling, self-control, obeying those in authority, proper language, cheating in school are just a few issues that can be highlighted after listening to the story of their day with their friends. Invite your kids' friends along on trips, drive in the carpool, and have your home be the place where they want to hang out. If it means installing table tennis, it's worth every penny to know where your kids are at night. Get to know their friends' parents as well. If you sense they have the same values or also go to church, do more things together as families. We found in backpacking with other families, our kids didn't complain much at all! Model hospitality by having potlucks with other church families – especially single parents who tend to get left out.

–Patti Francis, M.D.

• **Establish sound rules and consequences.** Be ahead of the game and not back-pedaling. Start when they are young establishing that mom and dad are the boss. Gather the data and listen carefully for their perspective before you pass judgment. Your anger can triple the consequences for your kids if you do not listen for a reasonable explanation that can bring you to a reasonable consequence.

• **Hold the standard of sexual purity.** Sex education starts in the home when children are preschoolers. The conversations should continue throughout grade school, middle school, high school, and young adulthood. What you say according to God's standard will go against the world your child lives in, but if one of your goals is for your child to have a healthy marriage, then it starts with waiting until marriage for sexual intimacy. And you are the most important person they need to hear that from! Lots of data support parental influence on a teen's sexual decisions. There is also research to support the relationship between cohabitation, sex before marriage, and lack of marital survival and happiness. Take every opportunity to turn off the TV, restrict the movies, veto skimpy clothing, and set boundaries for dating. Make sex worth waiting for. It's the best gift to give your child's future spouse – the gift of sexual purity. Take each child out at age eight and tell them how beautiful sex is in the context of mar-

Think of all the people you know who are hurting. It is often because they don't feel loved or because they are suffocating from anger over being hurt. It is critical that we pay attention to the way our kids relate to us and to others.

The best gift you can give your kids besides faith in Christ is a healthy marital relationship.

riage. You want to get there before anyone else and therefore be the authority on this subject. A great resource is *Teaching Your Children Values* by Richard and Lynda Eyre.

• *Most importantly, love your kids unconditionally.* Think about what your child's love languages are, as described above. Usually by grade school, you'll have a sense of how your child feels loved. Spend one-on-one time with each child and listen to their own goals and dreams. If they sense your complete love, when you disapprove of their behavior, it won't jeopardize their relationship with you. When they reach the teen years and want nothing to do with you, don't let them push you out. Connect with them on their level. Invite them to do something with you that they want to do. If you don't go away, they'll see that unconditional love shining through.

♦ENCOURAGE THEIR PHYSICAL WELL-BEING

As physicians and dentists, we know very well all the medical and dental problems that people can experience. We all want good health for our families and know intellectually what the right answers are. We encourage our patients to make healthy choices so as to live long and live well. Do we do the same for our families? Are we modeling healthy eating and exercise? The trends show we are still eating the wrong foods and gaining weight. We are getting less exercise in school and at home.

At the other extreme are the sports fanatics. Our kids rotate through sports all year and add music and Scouts on top of that, in addition to church programs. Many of us parents have been there and done that. Some children are so intensely involved in one sport that it consumes the family schedule with the parents driving them all over the state for sporting events, eliminating church and family activities. Parents live through their kids way too much.

Here are some things you can do to show your children how to balance their activities:

• *Model healthy eating and personal exercise.*

• *Eat dinner together as much as possible.* It might mean scheduling a few shorter workdays a week, but there are lots of studies showing the benefits of family dinner conversation being beneficial to kids' intelligence and well-being.

• *Let kids learn to cook at an early age.* They tend to be more interested in eating healthier meals if they are responsible for the choices.

• *Help your kids plant a vegetable garden* or their own personal fruit tree.

• *Let them pay for any junk food* out of their own allowance – just don't have it in the house.

• *Don't over schedule sports* and lead your kids to overuse syndromes and stress.

• *Take family walks together* – even in the rain or snow. It's more fun when there's a blizzard and you come back home to some hot chocolate.

• *Encourage sports that you can do as a family*, such as tennis, skiing, basketball, or soccer. We have an annual basketball game after Thanksgiving dinner and the winner does the dishes!

Discipline in eating and exercise is a lifelong task. We all fail at times and need to get up and try again. Your kids need to see that, too. It's okay to discuss how hard it is to avoid too many bad foods and to keep our exercise routine. But your persistence will show them how to do it for themselves for a lifetime. Remember, "Do you not know that your body is a temple of the Holy Spirit, who is in you, whom you have received from God? You are not your own, you were bought at a price. Therefore honor God with your body" (1 Cor. 6:19-20).

♦NURTURE THEIR EMOTIONAL HEALTH

Self-esteem has been the buzzword for the past twenty years or so, but attempts by our society to program it for our kids have been a terrible failure. Youth and adults are more emotionally unhappy than ever before. Teen suicide is much too common; drugs and alcohol still tempt our youth to cover up the pain. Without God, we will never have good self-esteem because our sinful nature will constantly overtake us. Romans 3:23 says, "...for all have sinned and fall short of the glory of God."

Here are some suggestions for helping your kids find their way to God's view of who they are in him:

• *Start family traditions* that your kids want to do every year, such as backpacking trips or other outdoor activities. During their teen years you may

Spend one-on-one time with each child and listen to their own goals and dreams. If they sense your complete love, when you disapprove of their behavior, it won't jeopardize their relationship with you.

Establish traditions for holidays and birthdays and other anniversaries. These remind them that they're part of a family that cares enough to share such things with each other.

experience some resistance, but more than likely if they had a great time sharing these things with you when they were younger, they'll want to join you again. Establish traditions for holidays and birthdays and other anniversaries. These remind them that they're part of a family that cares enough to share such things with each other.

• *Help them pursue their dreams and goals.* If you have a child who likes to draw, for example, you might provide opportunities to take classes or participate in a summer program that will support and develop that interest. Or maybe you'll have one who wants to be a wedding planner. You might help her connect with a wedding planner at your church or in another context. Perhaps your son wants to be a computer programmer. You should find him a Christian mentor in this field who can provide guidance and encouragement

• *Affirm those things about their character that you really like.* Perhaps they were kind to a new friend at school. Maybe they are generous in their giving to missions. Praise them for any attempt at a project, not just the grade they received. If they lost at sports, let them know how proud you are of their hard effort and good sportsmanship.

• *Tell them often that you love them* and give them lots of physical touch, even if touch is not their love language.

• *Be clear on your boundaries for them.* Kids will test the limits, but they feel more loved if there are some.

• *Dads, date your daughters; moms date your sons.* This will affirm their gender, which is something they should feel good about and someday will make them want to be attractive to the opposite sex.

• *Give them an allowance with portions for saving, gifts, missions, spending, and by middle school, for clothing.* As they learn what things cost, they will be proud of their ability to spend money efficiently and wisely. Their being generous also adds to their sense of self-worth.

• *By late high school encourage them to work.* Showing up on time and getting a paycheck teaches them what the real world is all about. Often we can afford what they need, but the earlier they learn to earn what they spend, the more they'll enjoy what they purchase with their own money and treat it with more respect.

♦Support their Education (Without Doing their Homework)

We all had to be on top academically to make it through medical or dental school. We had to push ourselves to the limit physically and emotionally to survive residency. Of course, we think our kids can do likewise.

It's very difficult for parents who are high achievers to remember that we once struggled with reading, finding our homework, or getting an "A" on every paper.

Our kids are not us. We must encourage them to be who God created them to be as they chart their course through the educational system. Here are some suggestions:

• *Model learning in your home* by seeking out knowledge when you don't know the answer. Have a good set of encyclopedias, other books, or Internet access.

• *Model reading as much as possible.* Read out loud at dinner or on vacations. Read a Christmas novel after dinner during Advent. Encourage your kids to read good biographies of great leaders. We all need heroes.

• *Attend their school functions* as much as possible to show your support.

• *Don't pay them for good grades* but let them eventually set the standard for themselves. It may take until college before they care. The more you pressure them, the more they will NOT care!

• *Do let them know there are privileges that come with doing their best* (not necessarily making straight "A's"), such as later curfews, driving, being on their own.

• *Limit TV, video games, and computer time* to one to two hours a day, or turn them off altogether. Take a stand and say "No" to poor entertainment. One couple allowed their kids to earn two dollars a week for book money when they chose not to watch TV during the week. They got hooked on reading.

• *If they struggle in school, get involved with finding out underlying problems* such as learning difficulties or ADD.

• *By middle school, students should start to be able to manage their own time for homework and sleep.* By high school, let them learn the hard way if they

> *Often we can afford what they need, but the earlier they learn to earn what they spend, the more they'll enjoy what they purchase with their own money and treat it with more respect.*

As our children grow to teens and young adults, we want them to be well-adjusted and happy individuals. They will have more success at work and in marriage if they grow up to be confident, assertive, and flexible individuals.

don't get it. Nagging them will only make them too enmeshed in your prodding to get it done. It's time to let consequences happen.

• **Have them visit a career/college counselor** in the first two years of high school to get a feel and a pep talk about what they might want to do after high school. Not all kids are meant to go to college.

• **Be involved with the curriculum**, especially the sex education material, throughout. Have discussions at home if you don't agree with the school's approach.

• **During the high school years, stay connected in whatever ways you can.** Agree that family members should know where other family members are. Parents should know who their children are with and whether adults are present. Cell phones can help! Drugs and alcohol are rampant! Don't fool yourself. They will be offered to your child.

• **Whatever your kids end up doing, cheer them on** and love them unconditionally!

As our children grow to teens and young adults, we want them to be well-adjusted and happy individuals. They will have more success at work and in marriage if they grow up to be confident, assertive, and flexible individuals. God has made them in his image and wants to transform all of us to become more Christlike. If we can yield our selfish desires within our marriages and families, the Holy Spirit will transform us into something beautiful. But it takes time and commitment for both parents and kids. It takes endurance through the tough times.

As busy practitioners, demands are ever increasing to see patients and fill out forms for people who may never remember your name. But your spouse and kids always will. Be there for them.

Our family backpacks in the Sierras every summer. If we didn't plan our trip well, train, trim down the baggage, and endure the pain of climbing a tough twelve thousand foot mountain pass, we'd miss the spectacular view at the top. On every trip we always take a group photograph at the top of the pass. There are many such pictures around our house and in my office. These remind us of the effort it took to get to the top. Our smiles reflect the painful steps and huffing and puffing. But they are smiles, and it's worth it!

–Patti Francis, M.D.

THREE QUESTIONS TO ASK YOURSELF

1. How committed am I to my marriage and spouse?
2. How much time do I invest in growing our relationship?
3. Am I faithful to parenting my children–protecting them from harm and teaching them to love God?

THREE ACTIONS TO CONSIDER

1. In prayer, focusing on the Great Commandment and Great Commission, write out all the commitments you have with work, church, community, family, and other. Ask God to direct you about where your priorities need to change.
2. Get out your day-timer/palm pilot and schedule your spouse and kids in for the next month with one-on-one time. Ask them what they need from you.
3. Discuss with your spouse what can help your marriage grow spiritually so you can minister to the broken world around you as a couple.

PRAYER

Dear Precious Lord and Savior,

Thank you for the gift of my spouse and my family. Help me see them through your eyes, with their unique personalities and giftedness. Show me how to love them unconditionally, as you love me. Teach me all about your forgiveness, so I might ask for it from them when I offend them and extend it to them when they need it. May we as a family become more like Christ and be a shining example of your grace and truth to a broken world.

—Amen

If we can yield our selfish desires within our marriages and families, the Holy Spirit will transform us into something beautiful.

Chapter 15

Our Colleagues and Communities

*I*was Director of the Family Practice residency program at the University of Minnesota and I had promised myself that I would NEVER bring up Christianity in any conversation or patient encounter unless I was first asked my opinion. I was determined to remain "politically correct" and inoffensive to everyone. I was also active in the Christian Medical & Dental Associations as a campus advisor and was the president of a Crisis Pregnancy Center Board of Directors, so most of my colleagues knew where I stood in my personal faith.

We had a social worker at our program who often sat in on teaching situations at the residency office to make sure the residents knew the various options available to them on ethical issues. He prided himself on creating "hot debates" so the residents would learn that many docs have different opinions on some issues.

One day as I was taking off my coat from teaching a noon conference at the hospital, this social worker was actively involved in an ethical discussion with one of my residents. When I walked in, he commented "Here's our religious zealot now." I entered the discussion and added my viewpoint.

After the encounter, I found the social worker in his office and asked him why he had identified me as a "religious zealot." I stated that I took that as an insult and found it demeaning. I told him that he could call me ugly or fat or a bad doctor, but I asked him to please NEVER insult my Christianity as it meant everything to me — and to my surprise — and his — I started crying.

Both of us understood the impact of my tears. He apologized profusely and said he truly "never knew my religion was that important to me." He never insulted me again and has actually used that encounter with the residents to teach them the importance of staying true to their own values.

–Ruth Bolton, M.D.

OUR COLLEAGUES

Representing Christ is no easy thing; secular people often watch to see if faithful Christians are "perfect." They accuse us if we are Christlike and they accuse us if we aren't. We know that perfection is beyond us, and yet we are indeed called to be holy in all we do. God expects us to "walk the talk" in order to make an impact on our world. We stand in full view of our colleagues, caught somewhere between their expectations as our fellow workers, our desire to please God, and our fallibilities as human beings. How do we ever get it right? Somehow God does it through us.

I found out years after my residency that two of my fellow residents had come to Christ with my witness having influenced their decisions. I was amazed because I had not fit in with them during the residency; I was too "straight-laced" for them. They later commented that they had envied my lifestyle and commitment. If I had known that they were watching, I probably would have blown it, but my innocent living for Christ paid later benefits in saved lives. How can I live my life intentionally so that my colleagues see Christ in me? In spite of my imperfections, how can I demonstrate character that draws my fellow doctors and students toward a closer relationship to God? These are questions we all need to keep in mind.

—Ruth Bolton, M.D.

WORTHY GOALS

If you truly want to be an impact player in relation to your colleagues at the office or hospital, it will help to keep these goals in mind: **practice excellence, demonstrate leadership, stand beside hurting colleagues, golf more, encourage, communicate accurately and honorably,** and **be ready with truth.**

♦Practice excellence

Colossians 3:23 says, "Whatever you do, work at it with all your heart, as working for the Lord, not for men." Or, to put it another way:

> "...don't do the minimum that will get you by. Do your best. Work from the heart for your eternal Master, God, confident that you'll get paid in full when you come into your inheritance. Keep in mind always that the ultimate Master you're serving is Christ. The sullen servant who does shoddy work will be held responsible. Being Christian doesn't cover up bad work."[1]

What platform do we have for sharing our faith if our colleagues don't respect us or feel that we are lazy?

When I was still director of the residency program, I often watched the new class of residents come in each year to see how they interacted and how they got along as the pressure of long hours working at the edge of their competence put them at odds with each other. The residents who covered the least work expected of them and those who would not rescue their colleagues who had a conflict with their call were often ostracized in the residency. On the other hand, the residents who went the extra mile were always cared for if they had a need. It seems like an easy lesson, but many had not learned it by the time they reached residency. I started teaching them to volunteer for call on Christmas right away and watch and see how their fellow residents treated them. They gained a great deal of respect among their colleagues.

I had the privilege of starting a Christian family practice clinic a few years ago and many of the doctors who now support our nonprofit clinic during our fundraisers are not Christian. From the beginning it was no secret that all of our doctors were born-again Christians. At our beginning we were hungry for new patients, so we volunteered to take as many unassigned patients as the ER would give us. At times, our work included physical examinations on elderly persons who needed to be in a nursing home. In order to help them avoid the inconvenience of a hospital admission, we would meet them and do the physical exam for the nursing home admission right in the ER. The social worker assigned to the ER noticed how we cared for the patients and started referring patients to us whenever he could. It did not matter that he was homosexual and Jewish and knew us to be professing Christians. Excellence and compassion was noticed in spite of his worldview

—Ruth Bolton, M.D.

> *The social worker assigned to the ER noticed how we cared for the patients and started referring patients to us whenever he could. It did not matter to him that we were professing Christians.*

Lazy Christian doctors suggest an apathetic God. We must do our best to act toward our colleagues the same way God has acted toward us so they can see who he really is.

♦Demonstrate leadership

I chose to be active in the hospital's leadership and was elected to be Chief of our Family Medicine Department. There are times I have regretted this decision, thinking I would rather spend my time working with Christian organizations. But doing things ethically and conscientiously has left a reflection of Christ even though I intentionally say little as a witness. A Christian leader is a servant leader and even though I was "elected" to be the Chief of a department, it wasn't a job that many people wanted.

—Ruth Bolton, M.D.

Our colleagues cannot follow us in God's way if we refuse to lead them.

Reflecting Christ in sacrificial service, with competence, speaks boatloads to our colleagues who are watching to see the Christ we follow. Maybe you should consider such leadership roles in your institution. People notice. Christ can be glorified.

Early in the first few years of my career, the doctors in my hospital voted whether or not the hospital should continue to perform abortions. I think we could have overturned the abortion vote if the Christian doctors had shown up to vote! Some of my fellow Christian doctors had gone to a drug rep dinner (and made a hundred-fifty dollars for attending instead of attending the medical staff meeting); some didn't want to close their clinic early and some were intimidated to make any statements. Our Chief of Staff leaned over to me the night of the vote and affirmed my previous public statements against continuing abortions. I asked him why he remained silent, if he believed as I did. He said it was because he was in leadership and "didn't want to sway the vote." Our hospital needed a true leader to stand up for what he believed in!

—Ruth Bolton, M.D.

How many children's lives would have been saved if that leadership position had been filled that night by a Christian doctor willing to stand up for God's truth? How many babies might not have died if Christian doctors had made that vote a priority? Our colleagues cannot follow us in God's way if we refuse to lead them.

♦Stand beside your hurting colleagues

Many times the hospital grapevine is a very vicious rumor mill. Have you ever considered volunteering to be on a committee that helps hurting doctors? Most hospitals have a confidential committee like that and most Medical Boards in the state do as well.

Have your colleagues ever asked you to be an expert witness for them in their malpractice suits? Usually, no one volunteers for such a role. If you believe that your colleague was not negligent, pray about it and step up to the plate.

Does that new doctor in town or in your practice have a place to go for Thanksgiving? Perhaps they are single or on call. Most singles have spent many a holiday alone, too proud to say anything to anyone.

In this same vein, consider mentoring a student. They absolutely love any time or attention you can give them. It doesn't have to be time-intensive; it can be a bike ride on your day off or a dinner once a quarter.

Our colleagues remember who stands with them when they are in pain. Be there with Christ and they will see him as he really is.

♦Golf more

One way I have found to mentor students and residents is to take them golfing or sailing. As a residency director, I would take my ten third-year residents on my sailboat for an afternoon to get an exit interview from them as a group. How could we improve the residency? It was a painless way to work! Besides that, I learned a lot about the students themselves, so much so, in fact, that I started taking the first-year residents sailing. I discovered that their personality sailing was very similar to their personality on call and in the office.

For example, one woman would "freak" when I gave her the helm and talk incessantly about how she was going to crash – the same thing would happen after her first few nights of call. Another man would take the helm and act as if he had been sailing his entire life – only to run us aground later. He was awfully confident in the delivery room as well.

I could find ways to teach them as I discovered where their strengths and weaknesses were. I was working while I was having fun. I think God wants us to have fun while we do his work. Our colleagues like to be around us when we are having fun. Everybody wins!

It took me over fifteen years to learn that my passion (addiction, possibly) to golf was honored by God. I have been able to interact with many colleagues through the annual hospital golf tournament. I don't think I would know most of the doctors at our hospital if I didn't golf. It has allowed me to interact with people much more comfortably. I've always said that our character is not made on the golf course, it is revealed! It's an incredible way to witness–all you have to do is count all your shots and not cheat!

–Ruth Bolton, M.D.

> *I don't think I would know most of the doctors at our hospital if I didn't golf. It has allowed me to interact with people much more comfortably.*

♦Encourage

Most doctors need encouragement. We work long hours; the pressures of paperwork, malpractice, and relationships are hard. Some of the best friends we have in medicine are the ones who have encouraged us when we've had one too many nights of no sleep and a too busy schedule. One way to encourage our colleagues is to build up their worth. It does wonders for your relationship with them and for their own confidence. Build them up in public, if possible. It has been said that most doctors often come out of conditional love backgrounds. Why else would we be willing to give up life in our twenties to study and stay up every third night? We come to believe that the harder we work, the more people love us. Doctors need encouragement.

Some doctors are encouraged by praise, others by humor. Many of us are too serious and should work hard to learn a good joke every week and then

We are mandated to hold fellow Christian colleagues accountable; we must do so biblically and honorably. Even more so, we must never denigrate the character of our colleagues who are not Christian by inaccurate communication or gossip.

lighten our colleagues' spirits by passing it on. Encourage, praise, tell jokes, and build them up in public. Think about what makes your day better and then do it for your fellow docs and students.

♦Communicate accurately and honorably

As I was starting our Christian clinic in Minnesota's Twin Cities, a wonderful P.A. (Physician's Assistant) had agreed to join me and had just resigned from an OB/Gyn group to help me start the clinic. After she had resigned, the only Christian doctor in that group took her aside and said that he wanted her to know something about me. He told her that he thought I was a good doctor and had a good reputation, but I was living a hypocritical life because I was a lesbian. By God's grace, my P.A. already knew me well enough to know that wasn't true.

The other doctor had made assumptions, like others may have, because the only other woman doctor that played golf in our hospital outings was lesbian – and guess what – we played a lot of golf together and often competed on the same team. This doctor had absolutely NO OTHER information that would make him think that. He could have destroyed me and my endeavor (God's work).

If he had really been concerned about my lifestyle, he should have confronted me personally rather than encouraging that kind of rumor. If we see that a Christian brother or sister is not living biblically, we must talk to them privately to make sure we have all the information, and then, either help them change their actions or defend them from rumors.

That doctor could have actually defended me had he come to me directly, instead of falsely accusing me. Thank God, I have learned that if anyone speaks falsely of me, my best defense is to live so that no one else will believe it.

—Ruth Bolton, M.D.

We are mandated to hold fellow Christian colleagues accountable; we must do so biblically and honorably. Even more so, we must never denigrate the character of our colleagues who are not Christian by inaccurate communication or gossip.

♦Be ready with truth

God tells us to be prepared to give an account of the truth:

> Preach the Word; be prepared in season and out of season; correct, rebuke and encourage – with patience and careful instruction. For the time will come when men will not put up with sound doctrine. Instead, to suit their own desires, they will gather around a great number of teachers to say what their itching ears want to hear.

They will turn their ears away from the truth and turn aside to myths. But you, keep your head in all situations, endure hardship, do the work of an evangelist, and discharge all the duties of your ministry (2 Tim. 4:2).

Over our years of practice, certain ethical dilemmas will come up time and time again. We need to anticipate them and be ready with an answer.

Our medical schools often teach that a doctor must be "values neutral" because of the position of power we have over the naked patient in front of us. It is not ethical to "force" our values on them. Indeed, we are not called by God to force our views on anyone; we are called to witness, to tell the truth as we see it. I have learned to confront values neutral thinking with the statement: "I'm not values neutral about smoking, or child abuse, or wife battery. How can I be neutral about abortion if I feel that a child is being destroyed?"

Do some homework so you know where you stand on important bioethical issues, and why; then use 1 Pet. 3:15 as your guide: "Always be prepared to give an answer to everyone who asks you to give the reason for the hope you have. But do this with gentleness and respect."

Remember that people without God's truth are blind and you may be the ray of light they need. Your colleagues will only hear rational arguments from a secular worldview if they do not hear good reason from Christians as well. CMDA is the best resource anywhere for literature, ethics statements, and information that can prepare you to present scientifically accurate and biblically based truth on bioethical issues.

"I'm not values neutral about smoking, or child abuse, or wife battery. How can I be neutral about abortion if I feel that a child is being destroyed?"

OUR STUDENTS AND RESIDENTS

I never meant to be a mentor; it just happened when this student asked if he could come to my office and discuss some things. He was young and bright and loved the Lord. He also was in medical school on the slow track because he had a learning disability. Our first meeting began a relationship that lasted four years. Each time he came, we walked through his study habits, his grades, and his emotional struggles. We walked through a romance where he lost the girl of his dreams. We walked through failed courses that had to be repeated. We walked through spiritual questions regarding the sovereignty of God.

My underlying message to him, repeatedly, was, "Seek with all your heart the will of God. Discover to your best ability whether or not he wants you to be a doctor. If you are convinced that he does, work with all your heart toward that end. Do not change directions unless he tells you to do so. Trust God. If you want his

One of our greatest responsibilities as Christian doctors is to help prepare our younger colleagues for the work God has in store for them.

will more than anything else, it shall be accomplished. If God then wants you to be a doctor, you will be a doctor. If he does not, he has a better plan for you anyway and your struggle here will help build you toward that plan."

There were many prayers, many struggles, and many disappointments, but they were all worth it when I picked up the phone and he said, "You can call me doctor."

—A Christian doctor

God's plan for this world is in our hands as he works through us. But someday he will take that plan from us and place it in the hands of those who follow. One of our greatest responsibilities as Christian doctors is to help prepare our younger colleagues for the work God has in store for them. Most students and residents will initially pattern their lives after graduate doctors whom they have admired. Who will they choose to mimic?

As Christian doctors, we must take seriously our responsibility before God to mentor students and residents. How do we do that when we often think: I don't have the time. I don't know how to mentor. Why would they listen to me, anyway? These sound like the excuses Moses gave to God at the burning bush. God wants most of us who have access to young doctors or students to train them in whatever lessons God has taught us along the way—even if that is only how to be a better doctor or a better spouse. Here is a simple plan to help you get started:

•**Understand mentoring.** It does not take special skills or training – just our willingness. It means spending time with someone else for the purpose of sharing insights, skills, and encouragement.

•**Find a young doctor or student whom you can mentor.** If you know of none, contact CMDA headquarters and ask them to help you find one.

•**Contact that student or doctor by phone.** You might say, "I am a Christian doctor here in town and would like to have you over for dinner and to get acquainted. If you are married you may bring your spouse." Set a date. If you get turned down, check back in a month or two. If you are still unsuccessful, seek another person to mentor.

•**Make your first meeting a social one** in which you discover who she/he is and help them relax in your presence. Focus your mentoring during that meeting on only one question: "How do you plan to protect and build your spiritual life during your training?" Follow that question where they wish to take you. End the meeting by offering to meet again next month. Set a date.

• **Prepare for the next meeting.** Check with CMDA regarding mentoring resources. Don't develop a plan, just discover what is available. The plan will develop as your relationship develops.

• **The next meeting should be more directed.** "How have you been doing with your training?" you might ask. "Have you been having any problems I can help you with? How are you doing with you spiritual life?"

This meeting should include a time of prayer and should help you develop a future plan, as in: "I'd love to get together with you every month to pray and share what we've each been going through. Would you be willing to do so?" Set up future meetings on a schedule that seems right for that individual's needs. Ask if they would like to look at Scripture or discuss some of the problems significant in a doctor's life, like money, time, family, or office practice. Arrange the time and place and put it on your calendar.

Mentoring should be deliberate and very individualized. For some relationships it will involve no more than a dinner get-together once a quarter. For others it may involve weekly or monthly Bible study, or an intensive review of books like this one. God knows what is needed. He asks our commitment. He will make the way plain and provide the time necessary. Pray seriously about this. You are a role model whether you wish to be or not. Why not make it intentional and God-honoring? Call someone today.

Mentoring should be deliberate and very individualized. Pray seriously about this. You are a role model whether you wish to be or not. Why not make it intentional and God-honoring?

OUR COMMUNITIES

When we read Luke 6:12-19, we see a day in the life of Christ (the Hebrew day runs from evening to evening), and we see a pattern for life we can copy for our own lives. We see Christ spending time alone with God in prayer (Luke 6:12) and then see him coming to be with his disciples (Luke 6:13-16). Then he and his followers (his community) go out and minister (Luke 6:17-19).

If we are believers spending time alone with God, he will lead us into a church community. And if we are spending time alone with God and in church community, he will lead us into ministry in our secular communities.

God has created us for a purpose and we will not find our wholeness and live out our purpose unless we fulfill that purpose in Christ. We have a mandate from God that leads us into a closer relationship with him, then with him to a circle of fellow believers, then with them into the world.

God has created us for a purpose and we will not find our wholeness and live out our purpose unless we fulfill that purpose in Christ.

God may call us into the community of the world in various arenas. Those arenas may be very specific for individual doctors, including these:

POLITICAL

How should we as doctors interact within our political community? Certainly we should do so with our vote. Our society desperately needs the impact of the Christian voter. We should study the candidates, understand the issues, and decide which candidates move our communities forward toward God's will—for the care of those he loves and the defense of his principles.

Some doctors are called beyond the vote to serve in positions of community service. Hospital boards, school boards, and charitable organizations need Christian input to accomplish God's best will for our communities.

A few doctors are called by God to run for political office. That calling is a vital one if God has clearly directed us. Political offices are dangerous for the Christian—persecution awaits the faithful and power corrupts the weak, but our communities and our country need doctors who can speak with their knowledge and experience about issues of education, bioethics, and healthcare with a spirit of grace.

SOCIAL

How should Christian doctors interact socially with their community? One of the problems of the Church is that we have isolated ourselves from the world and become foreigners with language barriers and social barriers between us and our secular world. Another problem is the opposite—some Christian doctors have so absorbed the culture of the world that there is no significant difference between their lives and the lives of unbelievers around them.

Yet we can be in the world, but not of it, if we:

- **Plan events with non-Christians.** Such events are critical to our witness and to our ongoing understanding of life outside the Church.

- **Spend time regularly and often with believers**—in worship and in fellowship. The world will fill the vacuum in our lives if Christian fellowship is missing.

- **Meet with non-Christians socially**, praying specifically ahead of time for God's presence in that event. That will not only remind us of our mission, but also remind us of our roots in heaven.

•**Enjoy ourselves socially.** Most people can identify an imposter who is present with a hidden agenda.

•**Never cross a moral line that God has drawn in his Word.** It is better to humbly and politely dismiss yourself from an activity, risking embarrassment, than to cross a line that God has drawn. Be careful, though, that the line is God's and not one fashioned by our religious culture.

HUMANITARIAN

How should a doctor impact his or her community for those who suffer? Whatever the motivation of the secular community in humanitarian efforts, if hurting people are helped, God is probably smiling. Christian doctors should be involved in secular humanitarian efforts as God's finger in the community because:

a. God wishes us to help those who suffer;
b. God's power is more likely to be manifested if God's people are present;
c. if we stand outside of such efforts, non-Christians despise the hypocrisy in our lives; and,
d. people are most open to the gospel when caring Christians bind their wounds.

Remember: Just because your church's name is not on the work doesn't mean that it is not God's work. Perhaps Christians need to make certain that our local churches are more active in such work and within it live out the person of Christ.

THREE QUESTIONS TO ASK YOURSELF
1. Should I take a leadership position among my colleagues when discussions of bioethical issues are on the table?
2. Do I respect and build up my colleagues so they might be brought closer to Christ?
3. Has God called me to some work in the secular community where he wants his presence visible through me?

THREE ACTIONS TO CONSIDER
1. Choose one colleague and pray every day for a year that you can bring him or her closer to Christ.
2. Take a committee position in your hospital or in your local government where a Christian voice matters.
3. Enlist in a project to help the suffering people in your community.

How should a doctor impact his or her community for those who suffer? Whatever the motivation of the secular community in humanitarian efforts, if hurting people are helped, God is probably smiling.

PRAYER

Dear Father,
You have placed me within a community of believers and non-believers. I some-times see elements of that community as something I can pick off the shelf and use for my own selfish interests and then put back up when I choose to be alone. Fill me with your sense of responsibility toward those you have called as a unified body to carry out your redemptive work. Let me not play "cowboy" with your great plan. Let me be a person of grace.

–Amen

NOTES:

1. From Col. 3:22-25, *The Message*.

CHAPTER 16

Our Testimony:

HAVING AN EFFECTIVE WITNESS IN A BUSY PRACTICE

*S*usan came to me with multiple complaints. Although her physical ailments were real, it seemed clear that there was an underlying spiritual problem. After addressing the specific complaints over a couple of visits, Susan began to reveal the real bane of her existence. Her marriage was failing. Despite the happy façade she created at work and church, she felt isolated and of no value.

When I suggested that God could help restore her marriage, she confessed that she had never felt that she really knew God. She knew about him, but she did not know him. She did not have the assurance that she was "part of the family."

After counseling with her pastor and me, Susan made a knowledgeable and intentional decision to accept Christ as her Savior and Lord. The change in her life was real. The subsequent joy she reflected so affected her husband that he too accepted Christ. As they matured, they became counselors to other struggling couples.

A marriage ministry was born in their church that was conceived in an exam room.

–Gene Rudd, M.D.

WE ARE SALT AND LIGHT

You are the salt of the earth. But if the salt loses its saltiness, how can it be made salty again? It is no longer good for anything, except to be thrown out and trampled by men.

You are the light of the world. ...let your light shine before men, that they may see your good deeds and praise your Father in heaven (Matt. 5:13-16).

We who are Christians are witnesses, whether we choose to be or not. As his followers, our choice, therefore, is either to be good witnesses or bad

"Be wise in the way you act toward outsiders; make the most of every opportunity. Let your conversation be always full of grace, seasoned with salt, so that you may know how to answer everyone" (Col. 4:5, 6).

witnesses. Jesus chose salt and light as metaphors for who we are in relation to the world around us. It is not a question of "if," it is a question of "what kind" of salt or light we will be. Good salt adds taste and preserves. Salt that has lost its saltiness is worthless – to be thrown out. Light that is hidden serves no purpose, either. But good salt accentuates the taste of godly things and makes people thirst for righteousness. And bright light illuminates his presence and work in our world. (We'll return to this part of the metaphor later.)

The apostle Paul wrote: "Be wise in the way you act toward outsiders; make the most of every opportunity. Let your conversation be always full of grace, seasoned with salt, so that you may know how to answer everyone" (Col. 4:5, 6). Paul is suggesting that our words and deeds be tasty and winsome to those around us. To be tasty, they must be full of grace, pleasant, and "seasoned with salt." Have you ever had fries or mashed potatoes without salt? Blah! Too much salt also spoils the flavor (as well as one's health), making both fries and our witness unappealing. But, salt in the right proportion makes potatoes irresistible–you eat some and want some more.

Our witness should be like that: tasty to a world that is hungry for flavor – a world in great need of the Bread of Life. Just as we seek proper salt balance in our patients, God calls us to be salt and light in just the right dosage.

The law of Theo-dynamics

Sometimes it's much too easy to forget that all our patients, all our staff, all our colleagues—in fact, all humans everywhere—desperately need to have what we have received by faith, outside of which they are all walking dead beings, as we once were. As the apostle Paul wrote:

> As for you, you were dead in your transgressions and sins, in which you used to live when you followed the ways of this world and of the ruler of the kingdom of the air, the spirit who is now at work in those who are disobedient. *All of us also lived among them at one time*, gratifying the cravings of our sinful nature and following its desires and thoughts. Like the rest, we were by nature objects of wrath. But because of his great love for us, God, who is rich in mercy, made us alive with Christ even when we were dead in transgressions–it is by grace you have been saved (Eph. 2:1-5; italics added for emphasis).

The foundational problem of the world is sin. Sin is the origin of all disease. Sin is the cause of humanity's separation from God. One way of thinking of sin is with a capital "S." Capital "S" sin began with Adam and our forefathers (and mothers). It entered the world, destroying the harmony man had with God and nature – bringing disease and enmity. It has been passed down to each of us in the form of our carnal nature, leading to our personal sins (small "s") that reinforce that destructive process in our lives and the world around us. Our bodies, minds, and spirits are doomed because we fail to follow the path God designed for us.

As a consequence, the scientific concept of entropy is applied to human nature. Things in this world move naturally toward disorder. We have cycles of tyranny, war, and strife. Our health progresses to disease. Our mental health tends to stress, depression, and confusion. Harmony goes toward anarchy. Wholeness goes toward emptiness. Death is inevitable. For entropy to be stayed or turned around, for disorder to become order, energy must be introduced into the system. Man has tried to do this on his own – with limited success in healthcare, but with no improvement in the human heart.

Our loving God, who created us for the joy of knowing us, ultimately provided the cure for the consequences of our sin. He provided the sacrifice, a blameless sacrifice, a sufficient sacrifice–his Son. Not only did Jesus show us how our broken relationship with God might be restored, he paid the price so that it might be possible. You and I do not contribute anything to this cure. God asks only that we respond to his offer of restoration through recognition and acceptance of Christ as Lord and Savior. Jesus Christ is the ultimate cure for all human misery. All those who believe in him have this assurance. If we are to tell others of God's great plan to restore their relationship with him, we must first be certain that we too have made this confession of faith in Christ, receiving forgiveness from and reconciliation to God. We cannot expect men and women to give up their lives to a cause that we ourselves do not passionately follow.

We cannot expect men and women to give up their lives to a cause that we ourselves do not passionately follow.

During construction of the CMDA headquarters, the project manager called me to schedule lunch to discuss "something." I assumed it was it was a problem with the project. After the meal and small talk he told me how God had used my witness to affect his life. He said, "I asked you to lunch just to tell you that I have decided to give my life to Jesus Christ." Wow!

–Gene Rudd, M.D.

Most of us would love to be part of such an experience, but even when our faith is real, we may fail to effectively fulfill our responsibility to be witnesses. Jesus used salt as a metaphor. As doctors, we understand this analogy. Salt balance is critical in our bodies. The beat of our hearts, the move-

*That same
grace of God,
working itself
out in our
own lives,
should reach
out to each
person he
loves, to each
person he sent
his Son to die
for, even to
those who are
not attractive,
even to those
who hate or
despitefully
use us.*

ment of our limbs, the processing of thoughts are each dependent on the proper balance of salt. A 10 to 20 percent deviation from norm can result in death.

Jesus said that his followers are salt. The problem with our witness is that we often fail at being the right balance of salt. Many of us know of fellow believers who are either hyponatremic (not salty enough) or hypernatremic (too salty). Maybe we are like that ourselves. We either fail to provide a witness or we tend to dump too much salt on others. In both situations, we fail to make the gospel more flavorful ("seasoned with salt"). Such salt imbalances are ineffective, even lethal, to our witness.

I recall a Christian friend in college. He had recently developed a passion for sharing his faith and therefore attempted passionately to do so with a fellow student. He was poorly prepared to share the message or to accept the response. Flustered when his witness was rebuffed by a fellow student, he responded by telling the fellow. "You can go to hell!" I wonder what flavor that fellow tasted after his encounter with my friend. It is not always easy to be effective witnesses to those whom Christ is seeking.

—Gene Rudd, M.D.

It is no accident that our salt balance is linked to the concept of grace. Grace means offering goodwill and mercy even though it is not deserved. It is the grace of Christ's sacrifice that provides us a way to restore the relationship with our Father. That same grace of God, working itself out in our own lives, should reach out to each person he loves, to each person he sent his Son to die for, even to those who are not attractive, even to those who hate or despitefully use us.

The underlying motive behind grace is love – sacrificial love that remains committed to someone even when there is no other reason to do so.

- Sometimes Christians attempt to witness from a sense of guilt or fear.
- Sometimes we do so because of peer pressure, as in a church outreach.
- Sometimes we even do so in a spirit of conquest or competition.
- But truly effective witness occurs only when it is prompted by love. If any other factor motivates our witness, it is misguided, and will probably be ineffective.

When love and grace underlie our witness, we have moved a long way toward the right balance of salt. When love and grace are missing in our witness, it is time to be silent. Mahatma Gandhi is reported to have said that he was attracted to Jesus and might have considered becoming his disciple–had it not been for Christians.

Perhaps you have heard of the great revival that swept through many college campuses in 1970. Many of the non-Christians on campuses admitted that the greatest obstacle for them accepting Christ had been the hypocritical lives of Christians! During the revival, when many Christians were moved to confession and repentance, a magnet of sincerity was created that pulled many non-believers into a relationship with Christ. Authentic Christianity does that. If authenticity does not mark your life, it is time to renew your relationship with God. In doing so, you will become savory to the world around you.

The Primary Barrier—Compartmentalized Thinking

Many of us as Christian doctors tend to compartmentalize our lives. Some of us are Sunday morning Christians only. For some, our witness is limited to an overseas mission trip once a year. We may not see the obligation to always make the gospel tasty. In Matt. 28:19-20 (often called the Great Commission) most English translations suggest an emphasis on the word *go*, as if Christ's imperative was focused on geography. This is reinforced by the following phrase that mentions all nations. Nevertheless, the command might better be translated, "Therefore, as you go, make disciples of all nations...." The emphasis is on making disciples as we go about our lives – all aspects of our lives. The practice of medicine and dentistry are not excluded!

Isaiah 6 outlines four steps in Isaiah's call to act as God's spokesperson:

1. **Awareness of God** ("I saw the Lord seated on a throne, high and exalted");
2. **Awareness of unrighteousness** ("I am a man of unclean lips");
3. **Atonement** ("your guilt is taken away and your sin atoned for");
4. **Invitation to service** ("Whom shall I send? And who will go for us?")

Isaiah's response: "Here am I. Send me!"

Preachers sometimes use this exchange to inspire the faithful to a life of foreign service. But where did Isaiah go? He did not go anywhere. He remained in service in the king's court. The change in his life was not one of location but of focus – a new willingness to faithfully proclaim the word of God. God's response to Isaiah's willingness to be sent was not to tell him to go to another place but to take the message of God to the people right where he lived.

The idea of being a witness right where you are counters the attitude among Christian healthcare providers in Western cultures that their workplace is exempt from God's requirement that we be witnesses.

Of course God calls some men and women to change their location in order to fulfill their role in his plan of redemption, but we must not shun our responsibility to help build his kingdom simply because our Maker chooses to keep us where we are.

The idea of being a witness right where you are counters the attitude among Christian healthcare providers in Western cultures that their workplace is exempt from God's requirement that we be witnesses. We hear the passage, "...you will be my witnesses in Jerusalem, and in all Judea and Samaria, and to the ends of the earth" (Acts 1:8), and we too often become focused on "the ends of the earth," forgetting our own "Jerusalem."

Of course God calls some men and women to change their location in order to fulfill their role in his plan of redemption, but we must not shun our responsibility to help build his kingdom simply because our Maker chooses to keep us where we are.

There are many wonderful role-models for us serving where we are:

♦While active in short-term medical missions, Steve Sartori does not limit his witness to his mission trips. The family practice he and his partners established in rural Kentucky has a reputation for being a light on a hill – providing quality care while pointing patients to Christ.

♦Rick Donlon is involved in missions daily, but the site just happens to be a few blocks from where he, his wife, and his children live in the inner city of Memphis. Rick and his partners established Christ Community Clinic, following the plan Christ gave to his disciples in Luke 9:2, "...he sent them out to preach the kingdom of God and to heal the sick."

Other Barriers Doctors Experience

Despite the medical literature, which demonstrates that spiritual issues are important to the health of our patients, doctors have wrongly come to believe that the promotion of spiritual health is not part of their job. How unfortunate – for both the patient and the doctor!

In a secular survey of 900 family physicians, the following reasons were given by doctors for avoiding spiritual issues with their patients:[1]

Lack of time	71%
Uncertainty about how to –	
Take a spiritual history	59%
Identify patients who desire discussion	56%
Manage spiritual issues	49%
Lack of experience or training	59%
Concern I will project my beliefs	53%
Difficulty using appropriate language	27%
Negative attitude of peers	23%

Patients, however, manifest a different attitude – a keen interest in spiritual things and a desire for their doctors to be involved in those areas of their lives. Data from several sources referenced in the *Saline Solution* workbook reflect what patients believe:

God loves me	90%
In the power of prayer	88%
God performs miracles today	85%
Physicians should pray with patients if asked	64%
Personal prayer heals	82%
Praying for others can help cure their illness	73%
Spiritual faith can help one recover from illness	79%
A doctor should talk to patients about their beliefs	63%

Our patients come to us trusting that we will do what is in their best interest. We need to learn how to transfer that trust in us to trust in Christ.

Of course there are unique challenges for the effective witness of physicians and dentists. Grace and professional ethics require that we not abuse our position of power and influence. God will not have it that way.

But fear of an ethical violation must not paralyze us. Faith and the practice of one's faith (religion) are associated with significant health benefits (80 percent correlation in literature reviews). It could be argued that it would be unethical not to encourage faith as a means to good health. Our patients come to us trusting that we will do what is in their best interest. We need to learn how to transfer that trust in us to trust in Christ.

Data compiled by the National Institutes for Healthcare Research (which is now called the International Center for the Integration of Health & Spirituality: www.nihr.org) reveal that 80 percent of medical research shows a positive correlation between variables of faith and religion and better health outcomes. Numerous studies show that people of faith, those who practice what they believe, live longer, enjoy better physical health, recover more quickly, and have more life satisfaction. If we had a pill with such wonderful benefits, it would be malpractice not to prescribe it!

While the evidence suggests that people of faith do have a healthier life in this world, the greatest reason for doctors to witness to their patients is eternal. Our participation in God's plan of redemption promises to bring rewards for all who listen and respond, far beyond the parameters of their physical existence!

As patients ourselves who have found the cure for our terminal spiritual illness, we ought to introduce others to the Great Physician who offers a cure to all! As doctors, the only way we can guide our patients to eternal health and life is to introduce them to Jesus, which most often occurs as a process rather than as an event.

The Process by which People come to Faith

Research shows that most people come to Christ through an incremental process – typically nine to sixteen steps. Perhaps more surprising is the pathway that most people follow to Christ. See how well you can guess. Fill in the blanks below with the percentages you think the Institute for Church Growth found when they asked people how they came to faith in Christ. Note that the actual numbers are at the end of the chapter—but don't cheat, now, try to guess first before you look!

Walk-ins (just showed up for church)	_____
Influenced by a particular pastor	_____
A church program	_____
Responded to visitation outreach	_____
Reached by Sunday school	_____
Responded to evangelistic crusade or TV program	_____
Influenced by family or friends	_____
Total	100%

Okay, now you can look.[2] Do the numbers surprise you? Though every process that leads others to Christ is important, we must ask ourselves where we should focus our efforts and resources. Notice the importance of the influence of family and friends. It is through these relationships that most people come to Christ in North America. "Men and women become interested in spiritual things when someone they know and respect takes the time and makes the effort to show them the way."[3]

Common barriers in the process

Let's go back to the concept of people coming to Christ through a series of steps. These steps lead them through barriers that each of us face when we are making significant, life-changing decisions – especially decisions that result in us giving up control.

The first barriers are *emotional*. Many non-believers in our culture have negative attitudes toward the gospel, the Bible, and Christians. This is often manifested as 1) denial, 2) indifference, 3) fear/mistrust, or 4) antagonism. These attitudes may result from bad experiences with hypercritical/judgmental Christians, those who lack integrity, or those whose message and lives are irrelevant. The first step for individuals with these emotional barriers is not a sermon; it is a person who cares for them.

The next barriers that non-believers must overcome to accept Christ are *intellectual*. People often have misunderstandings about God and his invitation through Jesus Christ. They may also want answers to some of life's perplexing problems. As Christians we can help them overcome these barriers by challenging them with the truths of God's Word – challenging them to consider the life and teaching of Christ. Sadly, most of us are not prepared to do this. It is even intimidating to many theologians. But the key is not having all the answers; the key is being willing to seek answers, sometimes together with the one who is asking.

The final barriers to hurdle are *volitional*. For many, the biggest issue is giving up control of their lives. Within each of us is a measure of pride and independence that is not easily given over to God. There is inertia and there are social pressures, each trying to deter a life change. This is where our persuasion, prayer, and the power of Holy Spirit are needed.

Underlying each of these obstacles (emotional, intellectual, and volitional) are spiritual barriers. Coexistent with each person's consideration of Christ is an intense spiritual warfare. Satan does not let go easily. People without Christ are spiritually dead. Satan wants them to stay that way.

Faced with such a challenge, it is important for us to remember that our success in witnessing is not determined by the outcome; our success is determined by our participation. Only God can raise the dead. We, as God's representatives in the world, do not have that power. But God, in his infinite wisdom, has chosen a plan of redemption that grants us the privilege of participation – of being on his team. We do not control the outcome, but we do control our willingness and availability for service.

As doctors, we have an awesome opportunity to be used by God for an eternal difference. Most non-believers in our culture will never darken the door of a church, read a gospel tract, or listen to a sermon on the radio, but they will get sick and have need of a doctor. God has put you right in the path of those who need his healing. We should anticipate that each patient is a divine appointment.

A missionary in the Middle East developed a burden for a people-group in a neighboring country. Despite his best efforts, he could not get a visa to visit that country. Then that people-group invaded his country with sixty thousand troops. As he was complaining to God about this offense, God revealed to him the opportunity to fulfill his passion of sharing his faith with these people. He responded to the opportunity, leading many to faith in Christ! Likewise, God, in his infinite wisdom, will lead someone to you whose heart has been prepared for your witness.

Sowing and Reaping

Remembering that only God can raise the dead, the most critical step for effective witness is our invitation for God to rule over the process and guide

People without Christ are spiritually dead. Satan wants them to stay that way. Faced with such a challenge, it is important for us to remember that our success in witnessing is not determined by the outcome; our success is determined by our participation. Only God can raise the dead.

Some doctors place "WIGD" on their charts or on their exam room doors as a reminder to first ask, "What Is God Doing?" before greeting their patients.

us to the right words for the right person. Our training has taught us that practice routines are essential for quality healthcare. Likewise, routinely invoking God's involvement is the most important element to success in the process of sharing the gospel.

In addition to starting your day in prayer, you can make it a routine to breathe a prayer just prior to greeting each patient. Ask God to show you what he is doing in that person's life and how you might become part of that plan (versus having your own agenda). Some doctors place "WIGD" on their charts or on their exam room doors as a reminder to first ask, "**W**hat **I**s **G**od **D**oing?" before greeting their patients.

Three concepts related to **respect**, **sensitivity**, and **permission** will effectively guide us around any pitfalls related to breaching ethical standards of care or abuse of power:

- **Respect** requires that our witness is properly motivated by love for each patient. It is love that seeks the best for them, even when there is much not to like about their attitudes or behaviors. We seek to do good for them because they are God's children. We extend respect to them because of the unmerited favor God extended to us.

- **Sensitivity** involves responding to each patient as an individual – not using a boilerplate witnessing tactic, but responding to individual needs and openness. This means adding just the right amount of salt to make the gospel tasty.

- **Permission** is hardly a new concept in medicine and dentistry. We seek our patients' permission for every intervention we undertake – sometimes implied, sometimes verbal, sometimes written. A patient who becomes stiff or distant when a spiritual issue is raised is not giving you permission. If there is doubt, we should clearly ask for permission before proceeding.

  You might ask, "Are you comfortable talking about these matters?" Or you might initiate a spiritual discussion by asking, "Since medical research shows such an important link between faith and health, may I discuss some spiritual issues with you?"

  There are many creative ways to seek permission. A pre-operative questionnaire might include the question, "Would you like the doctor to pray with you prior to surgery?"

Of course not all patients respond favorably to these types of questions, yet they may remain open to hearing more if the relationship is properly cultivated. Jesus reminded his disciples that the hard work of cultivation must be done before there can be a harvest:

> I tell you, open your eyes and look at the fields! They are ripe for harvest. Even now the reaper draws his wages; even now he harvests the crop for eternal life, so that the sower and the reaper may be glad together. Thus the saying "One sows and another reaps" is true. I sent you to reap what you have not worked for. Others have done the hard work, and you have reaped the benefits of their labor (John 4:35-38).

Sometimes cultivating hard soil and overcoming emotional barriers requires techniques similar to those used in encouraging change in other arenas of a patient's life. One important key is to include a spiritual history as part of your medical history. There are numerous examples of spiritual histories in the medical literature, but the method you choose to use may be as simple as asking these questions as part of the routine history:

*Is faith in God important to you?
*What impact does faith have on your life?
*How are you involved in your faith community?
*What do we need to know about your beliefs that might affect your health-care?

Signs posted in your office or clinic can also be an effective means of cultivation. Perhaps the most effective locations to display a sign in a medical or dental office is in the rest rooms! Some of our colleagues place signs on the ceiling over their dental chairs or exam tables. Here are some examples of messages you might wish to use:

Please let us know:

*If you are being physically or mentally abused. We want to help.
*If you might have a sexually transmitted disease. They often do not show up on routine examinations.
*If you would like to have someone pray with you. The doctor is happy to do so.

Sometimes cultivating hard soil and overcoming emotional barriers requires techniques similar to those used in encouraging change in other arenas of a patient's life. One important key is to include a spiritual history as part of your medical history.

Knowing how to cultivate the soil requires knowing something about the soil. Just as a farmer or gardener might obtain a soil analysis before planting, so a doctor can obtain a soul analysis before sowing the gospel by raising "faith flags." Faith flags are brief statements that identify you as someone to whom God is important. Here are some key elements of successful faith flags: they should take less than thirty seconds; they should flow into the natural conversation; they should identify you as a someone who believes in God but not as a member of a particular church or denomination; they should look for but not require a response; they should create opportunities for spiritual discussions for some patients; they should not be used to dump your whole load of salt on someone; they should not use religious jargon.

Knowing how to cultivate the soil requires knowing something about the soil. Just as a farmer or gardener might obtain a soil analysis before planting, so a doctor can obtain a soul analysis before sowing the gospel by raising "faith flags."

Here are some examples of faith flags for a variety of situations:

• "When I become discouraged, I find strength from reading the Psalms."
• "What do you think God is teaching you through this problem?"
• "Prayer is an excellent way to reduce stress."
• "My wife and I learned a lot about how to have a happy marriage through learning some principles taught in the Bible."

Use lay-level language

It is easy for us as physicians and dentists to overwhelm our patients with specialized words and information. The outcome can be expressed using the famous line from the movie "Cool Hand Luke"–"What we have here is a failure to communicate." Likewise we can fail to communicate the gospel by using specialized words and phrases. We may have grown up hearing these words, but many in our culture have not. Their use results in poor communication. As the apostle Paul expressed in 1 Cor. 9:19-23, we should modify what we say so that the words can be understood:

> Though I am free and belong to no man, I make myself a slave to everyone, to win as many as possible. To the Jews I became like a Jew, to win the Jews. To those under the law I became like one under the law (though I myself am not under the law), so as to win those under the law. To those not having the law I became like one not having the law (though I am not free from God's law but am under Christ's law), so as to win those not having the law. To the weak I became weak, to win the weak. I have become all things to all men so that by all possible means I might save some. I do all this for the sake of the gospel, that I may share in its blessings.

Below are some alternatives to a few of the words and phrases too often poorly understood by those outside the church:

sin	mistakes, shortcomings
lost	not knowing God, apart from God
gospel	good news God has for us
born again	become part of God's family
salvation	personally knowing God
washed in the blood	forgiven by the sacrifice of Jesus Christ
repent	turn your life around, go a new direction

Often, the way we express our words is more important than the words we choose. An article in *Psychology Today*[4] placed these values on effective communication: the words themselves–7 percent; tone of voice–38 percent; and gestures/body language–55 percent. Actions may well speak louder than words. We all know that our walk must match our talk. Similarly, our words need to be reinforced by the manner of their delivery. If we say our words with gentleness and concern, communication is greatly improved.

Be ready to sow gospel seeds when you sense that the patient (or any person) is open to a discussion of spiritual matters, or when they express interest in knowing more about your faith. This is an excellent opportunity to share a personal faith story. Faith stories are simply an expansion of faith flags. They are true short stories of how God, or a biblical principle, became relevant in your life.

For faith stories to be effective, they should be part of the natural conversation, take less than two minutes (don't try to preach a sermon), stay focused on God or the Bible, explain what it is like to be a child of God, avoid jargon, not push for a decision, not identify faith as a reason for not doing something, avoid attempts to convict (the work of the Holy Spirit) or condemn.

At age thirteen, I was a struggling "C" student. I worried about everything to the point that I was under treatment for a gastric ulcer. There was no apparent reason for the anxiety. I had a loving family that provided for me emotionally and physically. But I did not have the presence and peace of God in my life.

That year I realized that God loved me and had a plan for my life. The peace that followed resulted in the restoration of my health and the clarity of my mind. My homeroom teacher was so amazed at the turnaround in my grades that she visited my home to learn more. The story she heard was about a God who offers to bring peace into the midst of life's storms.

—Gene Rudd, M.D.

We all know that our walk must match our talk. Similarly, our words need to be reinforced by the manner of their delivery. If we say our words with gentleness and concern, communication is greatly improved.

As the Creator of time, God is also the redeemer of time. Somehow, in ways not always known to us, when we are obedient to his will, he provides the capacity and efficiency necessary to overcome our time constraints.

Preparing the Soil of your own Soul

Concern about time is one of the major reasons doctors give for not inter-acting spiritually with their patients. We are pushed from every side to be more productive. It seems an impossible task to provide quality, compassionate care within these expectations. We can't see how we can possibly add a new component to each patient visit.

The antidote for this concern is to remember that our God specializes in impossible situations. As the Creator of time, he is also the redeemer of time. Somehow, in ways not always known to us, when we are obedient to his will, he provides the capacity and efficiency necessary to overcome our time constraints.

This capacity starts when we invite God to rule over our lives each day. Begin each day and each clinic with prayer, asking God to quicken your heart and mind with love and wisdom. Ask him to make your spirit sensitive to the prompting of his Holy Spirit so that you might know when and how to deal with each patient. And ask him for the time necessary to make it possible.

When I first committed to share Christ with my patients, I made plenty of mistakes. One mistake was thinking that being a witness meant spending several minutes or sharing a sermon. When I decided that was not possible, the next mistake was waiting until my "guilt meter" registered so high that I responded by forcing a sermon on the next patient–ready or not. For some patients, this did not make the gospel very tasty. They were buried under a truck load of salt! But God was able to work even through those flawed efforts. Some hearts were changed–I was encouraged–and the Holy Spirit was working in my heart to show me a better way.

My next step in the journey was to learn to invite God to be part of my plan. He led me to others who gave good advice and encouragement. I began to see the importance of seeking to know God's unique approach for each patient. Prayer was the key. Not only did I need to start the day in prayer, I needed to invite God to preceptor me in each patient encounter. Again, I had to learn that such a prayer takes no longer than the time required to walk into a room. Prayers ranged from, "Help me, Lord," to "Let me see through your eyes."

I realized that I did not know what God was doing in that patient's heart, but he did. And he was willing to empower my feeble efforts. Sometimes this meant simply caring for the physical needs, providing encouragement, and raising a faith flag in hopes it would fall on fertile soil. Sometimes this meant showing kindness and establishing a basis for future spiritual conversations. Occasionally, it meant being able to recognize the root of a spiritual problem quickly and attend to a hurting heart.

God knew each need and how I was to be part of his plan. I needed only to follow. With each patient we should pray, "God, teach me what to say." Such earnest prayer results in the Great Physician being in charge.

—Gene Rudd, M.D.

In 1994, Walt Larimore (and his partners) were recognized by *Medical Economics* as having the "most efficient" family practice in America. Within the context of that efficiency, Walt was fulfilling his commitment to witness to his patients by asking for God's guidance for each patient encounter. As a minimum, he raised a faith flag with each patient. Time is not a barrier to God who desires to accomplish his will through willing servants.

Develop a "godly posse"

When your patients have need of a specialist, you make a referral. It is better for the patient. It is better for you. And it is a wise use of your talent and time. The same model applies to spiritual interventions. Not everyone has the same spiritual gifts. Not everyone has matured in the faith sufficiently to answer difficult questions. Just as healthcare is improved through a team approach, so can spiritual care be improved. You need a spiritual consultation team—what Walt Larimore calls a "godly posse!"

When I was building my spiritual consultation team, I visited several local pastors. Reactions ranged from sheer delight to disapproval. It became clear that not all churches are led by shepherds who are interested in evangelism. After evaluating each pastor's commitment to God, the Bible, and sharing Christ with others, I discussed how we might work together to meet the spiritual needs of my patients. It was clear that some were not prepared for this type of ministry. Because of the need for high professional standards, those willing but ill-equipped were not included.

The posse grew to include certain patients who combined spiritual maturity and experience through a particular illness that made them uniquely qualified to assist others through the same ordeal.

—Gene Rudd, M.D.

Your team might also include office staff, your spouse, lay leaders in the church, and when appropriate, Christian counselors.

Just as you require of your medical consultants, your spiritual consultation team must maintain the highest level of confidentiality. They, too, must honor the parameters of respect, sensitivity, and permission. Having training sessions for consultants will help them learn the rules of participation. We strongly encourage you to process these referrals using the same proce-

Another strategy that will help you manage time is to schedule follow-on appointments when a patient is in need of more intensive spiritual care.

dures as with medical consults. Generate a referral form for each patient to take to the spiritual consultant. The consultant (even if it is a fellow patient) should be expected to respond with an appropriate report suitable for the patient's chart. In addition to being good practice, this step adds validity to the concept of spiritual consultation. Last, but not least, use this consultation team for prayer support.

Another strategy that will help you manage time is to schedule follow-on appointments when a patient is in need of more intensive spiritual care. You might set aside one afternoon a week for catching up on paperwork and doing follow-up spiritual care appointments. There should be no charge for these visits—something not every practice would accommodate. However, God will lead you to a solution for how to meet the needs of patients needing more care.

Handling spiritual-care "emergencies"

A tension arises when an urgent need for spiritual care occurs in the course of a busy day. Do you let the office log-jam or do you ignore the opportunity? Here are some guidelines that will help you decide:

•Every ministry opportunity is not an emergency
•You are not called to meet every need—medical or spiritual
•For us, saying "yes" to someone means saying "no" to someone else
•God has called others to be part of his kingdom work

Therefore, you will need to rely on God's wisdom when deciding if:

•This a real crisis, or can it wait for a follow-up appointment or referral
•The moment is right, or if you should honor instead your commitment to those waiting

Develop a crisis management protocol, just as you have for medical emergencies. True life-threatening situations take priority. Sometimes you may have to call "911."

If someone called or came to our office wanting an abortion, we considered that a spiritual emergency. A life was at stake. Our crisis protocol went into effect.
—Gene Rudd, M.D.

There will be times in your work day when a spiritual crisis should take priority over your scheduled work. However, many time-consuming spiritual situations can be better handled by a follow-up appointment or referral.

Office decor can facilitate your witness.

There seems to be no correct answer for every setting. Some hesitate to recommend Christian art for fear that the messages on the walls will be different than the message heard from the staff's words and deeds. This type of hypocrisy is to be avoided at all costs. In some communities, Christian art or messages might turn away the very people you seek to influence. In other settings (e.g., the "Bible Belt"), Christian artwork and Scripture raise faith flags and provide opportunity for witness.

We have heard of mementos and pictures from mission trips turning conversations toward spiritual issues. Again, as did the apostle Paul, we modify our approach based on the audience.

Christian doctors also have other constraints to consider. Your employers or your partners may not approve of religious art. Remember, it is your job to be tasty to them as well.

Spiritual Prescription Pads

You can get dedicated prescription pads and a pocket reference guide to the resources available at the CMDA Resource Center by calling Life & Health Resources (1-888-231-2637). These prescription pads and pocket guides are free to doctors who will use them. The pocket guide describes resources that cover a wide variety of problems that our patients face, e.g., depression, cancer, marriage, parenting, etc.

Each resource has been screened by the CMDA staff and one or more Christian doctors. Just as you do when prescribing pharmaceuticals, you select the resource appropriate for the need, write the prescription, and instruct the patient to fill the prescription at their local bookstore or by calling CMDA's toll-free number.

We recommend that you follow up on the effects of this prescription just as you would for an antibiotic and continue to prescribe the ones that positively impact your patients.

Doctors can do only one of three things for their patients: 1) they can give them advice, 2) they can write a prescription, and/or 3) they can perform a procedure. We are well-advised to leave surgery on the soul to the Holy Spirit. However, advising patients to seek the things of God and writing prescriptions that lead them to an understanding of his truths are just plain good medicine!

Coworkers

Sometimes we overlook our opportunity to minister to our staff and coworkers. It could be argued that our obligation to them is greater than to our patients because we have an ongoing daily relationship with them.

We have heard of mementos and pictures from mission trips turning conversations toward spiritual issues. Again, as did the apostle Paul, we modify our approach based on the audience.

Sometimes we overlook our opportunity to minister to our staff and coworkers. It could be argued that our obligation to them is greater than to our patients because we have an ongoing daily relationship with them. Some need to know Christ. Others can be of valuable assistance in outreach to patients.

Some need to know Christ. Others can be of valuable assistance in outreach to patients. Value your staff and seek their input. Look for opportunities to pray together or hold Bible studies. Have your staff attend a *Saline Solution Seminar* or use the small group *Saline Solution* video series (1-888-231-2637).

Words of Understanding

Inevitably, when you have made the gospel tasty by properly caring for your patients, some will respond by lowering their *emotional* barriers. This stage in the process is called cultivation. As these barriers are being removed, we have the opportunity to address the next stage–the intellectual barriers. (Often there is overlap when dealing with these barriers.) These steps in the process are called sowing.

The *intellectual* barriers to knowing Christ are rooted in bad information. It is Satan's work to deceive minds. Guided by the Holy Spirit, it is our work to bring light into that darkness. This involves challenging an individual to consider the truths of the Bible, particularly the teachings of Christ. Again, some fundamental principles apply: respect, sensitivity, and permission; and see to it that the principles are applied with competence, character, and compassion.

We tend to take a deep breath at this point. We cannot imagine being asked a question we are not ready to handle. As doctors, we are supposed to have the answers. We feel uncomfortable when we don't. Sometimes this fear paralyzes us.

But it need not do so. We need only apply the same skills and procedures we have learned in healthcare. Just as the primary care physician refers for specialty care when the diagnosis warrants, we can refer patients for spiritual care. I have also found that one of the most important responses I can give to some with a difficult question is, "I don't know, but let's find out together."

–Gene Rudd, M.D.

Doctors may fail to address the intellectual barriers of their patients and colleagues for fear they are not prepared to answer tough questions, but most people who ask difficult questions are not doing so to win a debate point. While some may ask tough questions to frustrate you, for many, the questions and curiosity are real. Recognize this as fertile ground for sowing.

Winning the Argument or Winning the Soul

As people who are usually "right" we may find it easy to enter a competitive mode, wanting to win the debate, even if we are not successful in persuading the other person. But in relation to someone's soul, what have we gained if we "win"? What have we lost? While sowing the seeds of truth, we should remain motivated by love and guided by grace. Below are some examples of language that can either kill or encourage further discussion:

Killers:
- "It is a proven fact that . . ."
- "There's no question about it."
- "Only fools believe . . ."
- "That's ridiculous"
- "You are not serious, are you?"
- "If you believe that, you're going to hell!"

What makes the gospel tasty:
- "I hear what you are saying, but that raises a concern for me." (Respect)
- "Correct me if I'm wrong, but I see a conflict . . . ." (Sensitivity)
- "My perspective is a bit different. May I share it with you?" (Permission)
- "Have you considered this perspective?"
- "May I offer another opinion?"

While sowing the seeds of truth, we should remain motivated by love and guided by grace.

As with other steps in this process, the key is to recognize when the Holy Spirit has prepared the heart of someone to be receptive. Pray regularly for God to give you this insight. Pray for him to soften hearts. Pray for God to link you to others who can help in the process.

Proceed slowly, checking to be sure the person is understanding the path you are following. You may need to regulate the dose. Recognize that an expression of doubt is often a good thing. It may reflect that the person is giving the matter serious consideration. Allow the process to proceed at a deliberate pace – not pushing. Let the expression of doubt lead to further discussion and inquiry. Offer to directly share what God means in your life.

When faced with someone who is resistant to our witness, it is helpful to remember that our success is not determined by whether someone responds by accepting Christ. Our success is measured by our faithful participation in the process. In God's infinite wisdom, he gave mankind the choice to accept or resist his invitation. For we who are his children, God measures us by our obedience to effective witnessing, not the response of those to whom we witness.

Inherent in the sin of pride ("Pride goes before destruction..." Prov. 16:18) is the notion that somehow we are in control. God allows us to follow our own way rather than submit to him. The battle of good or evil, redemption or destruction is focused on this *decision of will* for each person. None of us begins in a neutral situation. The Bible teaches that we are all born with a

For those of us seeking a harvest, the key is persuasion — gentle persuasion. But while we get to be part of the plan, the Holy Spirit's work is ultimately required.

sinful nature that naturally rebels against God. This obstacle is called the volitional barrier. For our lives to be brought into a right relationship with God, we must yield our wills to his plan for redemption. As Christians, our participation in the plan of helping our neighbors overcome this volitional barrier is called harvesting.

For those of us seeking a harvest, the key is persuasion — gentle persuasion. But while we get to be part of the plan, the Holy Spirit's work is ultimately required. Here again, we need to bathe this process in prayer. Our persuasion must involve winsome discussion that invites someone to make a commitment to Christ.

While our Christian culture often portrays this process as culminating with a sinner's prayer, that model is not required by Scripture. The critical thing is that we believe in our heart and confess with our mouth that Jesus is Lord (Rom. 10:9). That decision of the mind and heart can come about in many ways besides kneeling at an altar.

Opportunity, Privilege, Responsibility

Our clinics, examination rooms, and hospital rooms are the most fertile mission fields in Western culture. While fewer than half the people in North America will ever darken the door of the church, everyone will become ill and have need of healthcare.

They will come to see us with the expectation that we will care for them. They come prepared to bare their bodies and soul, trusting that we will respond in their best interest. As those who have thirsted and found water, we have the obligation and opportunity to share Christ with those who are spiritually dry — living water from a well that will never run dry!

Prayer

Jesus said, "No one can come to me unless the Father who sent me draws him…" (John 6:44).

Repeatedly we have stressed the importance of prayer. From starting each day by asking for God's presence and power to work through your life, to breathing a prayer as you greet the next patient, to the earnest, committed prayer for a single soul, prayer is what leads to successful witness.

And prayer is far more than asking for "this" or "that." Prayer is that time when God wants to speak to a waiting, listening heart. It is the time when he will give direction and encouragement.

Prayer is what sustains us and keeps us on task as we seek to guide others through the many steps toward a commitment to Christ.

Take a moment to make a list of patients, friends, or loved ones you would like to see come to Christ. Begin praying daily for each one. Be open to what God will do through you to bring his will to pass.

"Men may spurn our appeals, reject our message, oppose our arguments, despise our persons, but they are helpless against our prayers."
—*J. Sidlow Baxter*

Now to him who is able to do immeasurably more than all we ask or imagine, according to his power that is at work within us, to him be glory in the church and in Christ Jesus throughout all generations, for ever and ever! Amen (Eph. 3:20-21).

Prayer is what sustains us and keeps us on task as we seek to guide others through the many steps toward a commitment to Christ.

THREE QUESTIONS TO ASK YOURSELF

1. How effective is my witness to my patients, staff, and colleagues? Am I too salty? Too bland? Or do people generally find me "tasty"?
2. Am I aware that people typically come to Christ via a process involving many, mini-steps? Do I now know how to use faith flags and faith stories to help determine where someone is in that process? Am I willing to let God use me to guide others toward taking the next step?
3. Does my walk match my talk? Am I committed to competence, character, and compassion as my interaction with patients is guided by respect, sensitivity, and permission?

THREE ACTIONS TO CONSIDER

1. Review the major points of this chapter. Make a list of the ideas you need to incorporate into your life and practice. Get more training by ordering the *Saline Solution* video series, a ten-part video and workbook course on witnessing in medicine and dentistry. Call 1-888-231-2637 or go online to Life & Health Resources at *www.cmdahome.org*.
2. Recruit others to assist you as you make changes. Perhaps they will include other Christian doctors, trusted assistants, your pastor, or your spouse. Use the *Saline Solution* video series for individual or small group training.
3. Pray! Ask others to pray with you. Start your day, each clinic, and each visit asking for God's perspective and help. Make a list and pray for ten people you would like to see become believers in Jesus Christ.

PRAYER

Heavenly Father, I acknowledge your Son as the Lord and Savior of my life. I ask for your presence, peace and purpose to guide me as I commit to make Christ known to others.

—Amen

NOTES:

1. *Journal of Family Practice* (Feb. 1999) 48:105-9.

2. Walk-ins (just showed up for church)	4-6 %
Influenced by a particular pastor	4-7 %
A church program	2-4 %
Responded to visitation outreach	1-2 %
Reached by Sunday school	4-6 %
Responded to evangelistic crusade or TV program	0.1 %
Influenced by family or friends	75-85 %

3. *Saline Solution*, p. 26.

4. Mehrabian "Communication Without Words," *Psychology Today* (Sept. 1978).

CHAPTER 17

The Critical Step

BY DAVID STEVENS, M.D., M.A. (ETHICS)
EXECUTIVE DIRECTOR, CMDA

I waited to write this chapter until I had an opportunity to read the rest of the book. Like you, my thinking has been stimulated and my heart has been challenged. I hope you have grasped a clear vision of what it means to practice by the Book.

Vision is great—but vision without personal change is like a car without gas. Such a car may be pleasant to look at but it won't get you anywhere! In fact, you would just be frustrated by it every time you had to maneuver your bicycle around it on your long trip to work! You would be happier if you didn't even know the automobile existed.

You know now that there is a better way to practice medicine: a way that will provide personal fulfillment, bless your staff, and minister to your patients. Yet to really benefit from what you have read, you have to change. Knowledge of what it means to be a Christian doctor, what it means to have a uniquely Christian practice, how to express compassion, and the importance of caring for the poor can be of academic interest or it can influence your new practice style. It's up to you.

Perhaps you have already incorporated some of the principles you've just read about into your practice. I hope so. Still, I don't know a Christian physician or dentist who would get a perfect score on practicing by the Book, especially me. There are always areas where we need improvement.

All of us still have work to do.

Perhaps you are a professional student grinding your way through books, classes, exams, and rounds. You may be longing for the day when you will actually begin to practice in a way that honors Christ. Many Christian doctors have gone before you with such a longing, only to wake up some time later, pick up the pieces of their mistakes and realize that their practices have become just like every secular practice around them. They have dis-

Change is not easy. We are naturally comfortable staying where we are—swept along by the current of the status quo. It takes effort to swim upstream, to become all that God desires us to be as Christian doctors.

covered that if Jesus showed up as a patient, he wouldn't see any difference in their practice from that of the non-Christian doctor next door. The medical system sucked them in. They didn't fight hard enough against the flow. Now is the opportune time to decide to do it right the first time around. Now is the time to determine to be different.

Or, you may already be a doctor in clinical or academic practice. Wherever you are in your training or career, be encouraged that you've taken an important first step. You've read this book. You're standing at the starting line. It is time to get in the race. Now is the time to change.

Change is not easy. We are naturally comfortable staying where we are—swept along by the current of the status quo. It takes effort to swim upstream, to become all that God desires us to be as Christian doctors. In order to change we have to overcome inertia, busyness and other priorities. That takes vision and determination – a desire to be different that can only grow out of discontent with where you are now. You have to believe that there is something better and you must be determined to achieve it.

Living your life as a Christian doctor requires work but it is worth the effort, at a minimum because it will make you more fulfilled and happy, but all the more because it will please God and cause him to delight in you. Such a life is worth striving for because it will let God use you better to build his kingdom. You can become the doctor that God designed you to be—but it requires change.

I am no stranger to change. When I arrived at the mission hospital where I served for eleven years, we were averaging 180 percent occupancy for the year. How is that possible? We put two or three patients in a bed with the family members sleeping on the floor. The hospital only had electricity part of the day and none at night. I was putting three to five cut downs a day into kids with dehydration and shock from gastroenteritis caused by the contaminated river water they were drinking at home. We got them better, but gave them the same bacteria-laden untreated river water from our faucets that they got at home since we didn't have a water treatment system. Half of the patients in the hospital had easily preventable diseases and basic public health measures would have averted half our deaths.

Ours was the main hospital for 300,000 people. I had my hundred thousand patients and the other two doctors each had their hundred thousand! We were caught in a vortex of a never-ending flood of patients. The only way out of this whirlpool was a new vision and determination.

How were we going to implement change when we couldn't even keep up with our daily workload and call schedule? The alternative was even worse. We could continue to just barely keep functioning and gasping for breath when our heads got above water while people needlessly died. Something had to change.

We looked at our resources, reprioritized our time, and began to strategically plan. It took extraordinary effort. We started with a community health program using volunteers to teach better health practices to their neighbors, treating the ten most common diseases, and sharing the gospel door to door. It was remarkably successful. We developed a master plan for the hospital and expanded from 125 beds to 300 beds. We were the first mission hospital in Africa to computerize our billing, finances, and databases. We drew up a mission statement, wrote a new hospital constitution, and developed a new organizational structure. We built a 320-kilowatt hydroelectric plant to provide cheap twenty-four-hour electricity. With our savings in generator fuel costs, we started a nursing school to train staff. We started a chaplaincy training school, expanded our spiritual ministry, and taught local pastors how to follow up and disciple new converts. Looking back, it is amazing to remember what God did and to learn from my experience all that is required to bring about worthwhile change.

STEPS TO CHANGE

1. The first step toward change is an **intense discontent** with how things are now. If you wish to change, you must evaluate your present life and find yourself unhappy with the status quo. You must be determined to move from where you presently are, and you must be willing to risk change. What areas in your life stood out as distasteful or underdeveloped as you read this book? Where has God pointed in your life and said, "That is not my best plan for you"? Choose three such areas of discontent and plan to make those your areas of improvement.

2. The second step is to **develop a vision** of something better. Now that you have read stories of how your practice could be and learned principles that you can apply to your life and practice, you can envision a different picture of medical or dental practice. Continue to add fuel to the flame that has been lit. Tend the fire of your vision by visiting good Christian practices and learning from them. Start a correspondence with distant doctors who can mentor or give you advice. Learn from others' experience to speed your learning curve.

When I started our community health program in Africa, I knew little about adult education techniques, motivating and managing volunteers, or doing outcome-based research. So I found people who did. We put together a

The first step to change is an intense discontent with how things are now. If you wish to change, you must evaluate your present life and find yourself unhappy with the status quo.

Now you need to lay out a plan to follow toward that change. Look at your own life and practice as objectively as you can.

survey instrument and visited over a dozen programs in Kenya to find out what was working and what wasn't. We copied their successes. We identified their problems and tried to design our program to avoid them. We collected forms, teaching materials, and anything we could get our hands on to guide our thinking and lessen our workload. It was the most valuable thing we did. It helped us to flesh out our vision until the picture was clear. We did the same for others when we became one of the most successful programs on the continent. Doctors and nurses from over twenty countries came and visited our program to help refine their strategy and to get materials to help lessen their workload.

You can do the same with your areas of weakness. Find the doctors you know who are strong where you are weak. Meet with them and catch a vision of how you can change.

3. The third step of change is to **plan**. You have identified your areas of life and practice that most need changing. You have caught the vision of how you can be different; how you can be more like the Great Physician. Now you need to lay out a plan to follow toward that change. Look at your own life and practice as objectively as you can. What are you doing well and where are the biggest problems? Is your problem time management, or staff morale, or finances, or spiritual outreach to patients, or family difficulties? You will not change unless you lay out the steps to do so. This book will help you in some areas. Good doctor mentors will help you as well. You may need pastoral or professional counseling in other areas. Take the three areas you have chosen; develop a plan for each on a separate sheet of paper; put the plan where you can't forget it; and then, you'll be ready to get started.

How do you change if you are part of a multi-doctor practice? If you have partners in your practice, you need to draw them into the process. They need to realize the need for change and you each need to share a common vision. Meeting for discussion, prayer, and planning can facilitate this. Such meetings should be held when you are most likely to have an undisturbed hour together. Some doctors meet for an early breakfast. Other practices have scheduled a mini-retreat in order to get a lot done quickly. If possible, have all the partners involved. To use your time wisely, draw up an agenda and allocate time to each section. Keep the discussion moving and have the goal of developing a list of action items that you can begin working on. Some groups have divided and conquered. One doctor investigates staff morale and works on a plan for the group while another focuses on another area, like finances. Individuals do most of the legwork and then bring their findings back to the group for input and refining.

If you don't have the time or desire to do this yourself, you may need an outside facilitator such as a Christian practice consultant who can do the evaluation and help you establish a plan. A consultant can also share the experience of many other practices with you. It will cost something, but the result is a quicker process and better results. At www.cmdahome.org you will find a list of consultants who have been recommended by CMDA members.

Even if you use a consultant, you and your partners are the only ones that can accept or modify the change plan, prioritize action items, and get the ball rolling. You are the key to personal and practice improvement. Ask God for wisdom, strength, and guidance and then lead people to change.

At some point, you will also need to get your support staff involved in planning the change. This will make every change that much easier because they have already bought into the vision and have helped design the strategy before implementation.

Set a completion goal and intermediate assessment points. Often this is easiest when a time line is posted for everyone to see. It should show who accomplishes what by when. If you don't do this, you will get busy with the urgent and forget to work on the essential.

4. The fourth step in change is **action**. Dag Hammarskold was Secretary General of the United Nations when he died seeking peace in the Congo in 1961. This man of God wrote, "In our era, the road to holiness necessarily passes through the world of action." It is the same for our individual lives now as it was for the world in 1961. We cannot simply wish and plan to be different; we must take action. Make sure you get started. You don't have to do everything at once; begin with one of the three areas at the top of your priority list. Then, take the first step.

At your assessment points, evaluate your progress, roadblocks, and possible solutions. Use these times to *hold yourself and other participants accountable*, to *publicly recognize* those who have reached their goals and to *motivate* and advise those who are dragging behind. It is often not what you recognize or reward people with, but how you do it that counts. Rewards should have meaning and be given in front of significant others. Rewards that can be displayed will continue to have significance in the person's life. Isn't that why you keep your medical school diploma on the wall and golf trophies on your display shelf?

In my mission setting, one of the keys to motivating whole communities to change their health practices was our healthy home certificate, which had emblazoned on it, *Kichamege in Ga* – "we are well in our home."

"In our era, the road to holiness necessarily passes through the world of action."

–Dag Hammarskold

*In
implementing
personal
change,
a mentor or
friend is
critical in
accomplishing
your goals.*

If a family changed five health practices such as boiling their water, building a latrine, and having their children immunized, the community health worker, a health committee member, and the assistant chief would come and inspect their home. If they passed inspection, the chief would call them up in front of everyone at the next village meeting, praise them, and give them a certificate with a red ribbon and big gold seal. They would put the certificate on the wall in their hut and their neighbors would come by and ask, "When did you graduate from the University? How did you get that beautiful certificate?" They would explain about changing five health behaviors. By the third year of our program, we were giving out 8,000 certificates a year. They were rewards, visible recognition, advertisements, and a great motivation to change.

To motivate change in the communities around our hospital in Africa, we worked at motivating people at every level. We set standards for our national supervisors and those that reached them were taken with their wives on a special overnight trip to the game preserve. Most of them had never seen a lion or elephant and each of them was so motivated that everyone exceeded the standard.

I like designing two types of reward/recognition systems. In one, whoever does the best gets recognized and in the other, everyone who meets the minimum level of achievement is recognized. That way, more people participate and change more readily takes place.

Just as we did in Africa, you should find ways to reward those who help you in your move toward a practice that most honors our King.

Accountability is as important as motivation. Most people need it. Medical school tests were assessment points that caused each of us to stay up late studying the night before. In implementing personal change, a mentor or friend is critical in accomplishing your goals. I recently decided to lose some weight, so I called my brother in another state and challenged him to compete with me in this endeavor. Whoever lost weight first gave a specified reward to the other. I thrive on competition and I knew I would work hard to win.

People like to compare themselves to others to make sure they are performing well. In medical school, our professors posted our test grades on a bulletin board with our ID number. After I looked at my grade, what did I do next? Of course, I looked to see what everyone else had gotten on the test! Was I in the middle of the class or at the top? All of us compare ourselves with others. That is why periodic job performance reviews are so important. They let staff know that they are doing their job and doing it well. You can do this in a practice, too, with departments or individuals competing in getting something done or improving quality. Not only can you set up competition between individuals, but against standards. For example, set a standard for how quickly staff members move patients from the front door to sitting in the exam room. Monitor the results and then recognize and/or reward those that exceed the standard consistently.

Self-discipline and *persistence* on our part are important because change is hard to implement. Drug reps know that it takes several visits to get you to change your prescribing habits. You cannot change your own habits or those of others without the discipline of monitoring results and modifying your strategy as necessary to get where you want to go. Change is mainly about persistence until you and your staff establish new systems and habits.

After that it will start to come naturally, but don't stop when you think you have arrived. Continue to discuss ways to improve and make things better. As it is in our Christian walk, your practice will never really "arrive" while you work with God on this side of heaven. It will never be perfect. There always will be better ways to do everything. That is especially true with the world constantly changing. The method that worked five years ago may no longer be the best way to do things.

You can "practice by the Book." Others have and you can, too. The vision may seem too formidable, but you are not alone. Fix your eyes on your goal. Then break it down to achievable steps and get started. You will not be satisfied with your walk with Christ or your practice until you do. The good news is that you already have a model and you have someone to help you do it. Christ himself will lead the way. Then you will lead others. May God empower you to follow his lead so that we may all "practice by the Book" and change the face of healthcare into the image of Christ.

Dear God,
You have placed me in this world as a doctor with a plan for my life. I have read this book and seen the possibilities. I now hold this book up to you. Take from it what you choose for my life and begin the change in me. Give me the insight and determination to follow through and become the Christian doctor you have created me to be–by your power, with your wisdom, and for your glory.

–Amen

You cannot change your own habits or those of others without the discipline of monitoring results and modifying your strategy as necessary to get where you want to go.